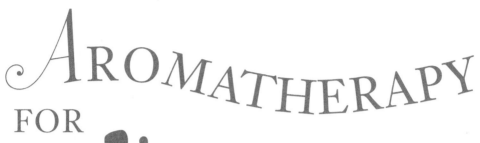

AROMATHERAPY FOR Lovers

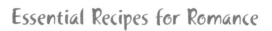

Essential Recipes for Romance

by Tara Fellner

JOURNEY EDITIONS
Boston • Rutland, Vermont • Tokyo

This edition published in 2001 by Journey Editions, an imprint of Periplus Editions (HK) Ltd., with editorial offices at 153 Milk Street, Boston, Massachusetts, 02109.

Library of Congress Cataloging-in-Publication Data in Process
ISBN: 1–58290–046–9

NOTE: The aromatherapy oils and instructions given in this kit are not for medicinal use. Please refer to the safety information on page 145 before applying any of the recipes or blends included in this kit. Neither the author nor the publisher are responsible for any injury that may occur through following instructions in this book.

Illustrations by Rebecca Daw

Distributed by

USA	Asia Pacific	Japan
Tuttle Publishing	Berkeley Book Pte Ltd	Tuttle Publishing
Distribution Center	5 Little Roas #08–01	RK Building, 2nd Floor
Airport Industrial Park	Singapore 536983	2–13–10 Shimo-Meguro,
364 Innovation Drive	Tel: (65) 280-1330	Meguro-Ku
North Clarendon, VT 05759-9436	Fax: (65) 280-6290	Tokyo 1530064
Tel: (802) 773-8930		Tel: (03) 5437-0171
Tel: (800) 526-2778		Fax: (03) 5437-0755
Fax: (802) 773-6993		

3 5 7 9 10 8 6 4 2 1   06 05 04 03 02 01

Printed in the United States of America

Contents

iii

ONE

Aromatherapy for Lovers: The Basics

I

A Brief and Fragrant History of Love; Smell Perception, or Why There
Are No Perfumes in Outer Space; The Limbic System: "Pleasure Central";
The Smell of Love and the Point of Perfume; The Big "O," or Love,
Orgasm and Oxytocin

v

Preface and Acknowledgments

Of all the mysteries that enchant us,
love is my favorite.
DIANE ACKERMAN, *A Natural History of Love*

WHAT IS LOVE? Where does it come from? Where does it go when it fades away? These are questions that have occupied humankind for thousands of years. You'd think we'd have some answers by now! Yet the mystery remains for each human being to unravel anew. Every heart is an uncharted wilderness, a new frontier. To love, and to be loved, requires above all a sense of adventure, a capacity for wonder, and a willingness to put up with substandard accommodations occasionally along the way.

So many people I talk to are frustrated in their pursuit of love. Those who have found romantic love struggle to keep it alive amidst the drudgery and mundane concerns of everyday life. One of the most common complaints I hear among my contemporaries is the feeling that we are on the front lines of the gender wars. What does it mean today to be a man, to be a woman? Who plays what role when, and for how long, and with what degree of enthusiasm? Who does the dishes?

A recent article in a national magazine exploring the reason so many highly successful, highly attractive professional men and women in the prime of life remain single, intimated that it was because they had no real need for a mate. With our nation's greater than 50% divorce rate, romantic expectations of "happily ever after" can seem far out of reach.

Do men and women still need each other? I think we do! While it takes some special effort to create a haven in which love can thrive, the rewards are great. Aromatherapy and the use of essential oils can contribute to a smoother, happier, more intimate and exciting love relationship. Everything you need to begin can be found right here.

This book is intended as a tool to increase your enjoyment of love, and your lover. But it's not enough just to read it. You have to practice, too! The kit includes three true aromatherapy massage blends, formulated with authentic essential oils that have been used traditionally by lovers for thousands of years for their aphrodisiac effects: "Clouds and Rain," which contains pure essence of jasmine and is named for the translation of the Chinese expression describing simultaneous orgasm, "Ecstasy Rub," based on ylang-ylang, and "Rose Petal Caress," made with rare and precious rose Bulgare.

Do they work? The publisher of a popular aromatherapy newsletter, overheard by a stranger while she was discussing the aphrodisiac properties of rose, put it this way: "He asked me if I really believed in aphrodisiacs. I simply answered, 'I didn't used to.'"

This book has been a great deal of fun to research and to write, and I give my never-ending thanks to Michael Kerber of Charles E. Tuttle Co. and Ron Schultz of

Learning Arts Publications for the opportunity to engage in such pleasurable work! Thanks also to the rest of "the gang" at Learning Arts, and Terry Duffy and David Skolkin. My undying gratitude to Eric Boles for wearing both parental hats for Maggie and Nick while I pushed to finish.

Thanks also to my teachers, Michael Scholes, Dr. Kurt Schnaubelt, and John Steele, for sharing their knowledge of essential oils and for their ongoing research and inspiration. Lucia Edna Lopez and Janet Celia Lopez, Debbie Gerlock, Debra Kay and Greg Evans, Carol Corio, and Eugenia Melissaratos, thanks for your help and support. This book also would not have been possible without the pioneering work of the women who have contributed so much to the popularization of aromatherapy, and from whose greater wisdom I have borrowed, both conceptually and in spirit. I would like to thank Marguerite Maury, Danièle Ryman, Patricia Davis, Valerie Worwood, Annemarie Buhler, Jane Kennedy, and Tara Kamath (to name but a few!) for their energy, ideas, and perseverance in the day-to-day work of making the joys of aromatherapy accessible to a world that so desperately needs it.

ONE

Aromatherapy for Lovers:
The Basics

To love is to return to a home we never left, to remember who we are.
SAM KEEN, *The Passionate Life*

A Brief and Fragrant History of Love

EROTIC LOVE IS PRIMAL AND ANCIENT, as integral to being human as our capacity for speech and our penchant for creating tools and technology. Once upon a time, before we learned to "drive our bodies with the brakes on" (as Tantric teacher Margo Anand so succinctly puts it), erotic experience was the focus of life and a way of connecting with the divine. Our earliest myths and religions deified erotic love, explaining the origin of life and the universe as the interaction of divine sexual energies. The coming together of these potent, life-giving forces was reenacted during ritualized lovemaking, the earliest form of worship.

To ancient peoples, everything in Nature was alive with spiritual and sexual possibility. Human sexual energy was believed to prime the generative functions of the Earth and Sky, ensuring the fertility of livestock and crops that was necessary for early cultures to flourish. Rain was a fertilizing fluid that fell from the sky god to impregnate the Earth. The sexual vigor and fecundity of ancient gods and goddesses led to their being symbolized in the forms of prolifically breeding animals such as bulls, goats, cows, and horses. Music and pageantry exalted consciousness and stirred the senses. Because they were part of worship, sex, incense, and perfumes were sacred. In the old Germanic languages, the word *lust* was synonymous with religious joy.

The origin of the word *love* can be traced back through time to the Sanskrit *lubhyati*, he desires. The word *erotic* is a gift from the ancient Greeks, who believed that Eros, or Love as pure generative and co-creative power, permeated all that existed. In the beginning, according to the ancient Greek playwright Aristophanes,

> Black-winged Night
> Into the bosom of Erebus dark and deep
> Laid a wind-born egg, and as the seasons rolled
> Forth sprang Love, the longed-for, shining, with wings of gold.

Love (Eros) is born from confusion and darkness, hatching miraculously from an egg laid in Erebus, the house of Death. Love then creates Light and Day and goes about illuminating existence with its torch, playfully shooting the Universe full of holes with arrows of desire. Eros is the matchmaker who joins Heaven and Earth. From Love comes Light, Life, and Being, yet its parents are Darkness and Death.

In later mythology, Eros is personified as Cupid, son of the love goddess Venus (known to the Greeks as Aphrodite). Familiar to us as a winged cherub holding a bow and arrow, Cupid is a perpetual child who, to his mother's continual frustration, won't grow up. Kama, the ancient love god of India, is also an archer with a quiver full of flower-tipped arrows with which he pierces the heart through the senses, symbolic of the powerful connection between fragrance and romance.

Have we changed all that much in the last few millennia? Not when it comes to love. Aristophanes' words are nearly two and a half thousand years old, yet his description of falling in love is just as apt today: the initial, winged rush of feeling, the sensation of sudden and complete illumination. Civilizations rise and fall, but Love continues to pierce us with the same bright, scented arrows, transforming existence in showers of golden light.

The association of love and fragrance is closely interwoven with human history, predating Roman times. Many Roman customs and festivals were borrowed from even older Etruscan, Phoenician, and Greek traditions, and some, May Day, for example, survive into the present day. As children, we used to hang baskets of flowers (hard to come by on the first of May in Wisconsin!) on the doors of friends' and neighbors' houses, ring the doorbells, and run away. Little did we know we were commemorating an ancient fertility rite, Floralia, during which the Romans honored Flora, goddess of spring and flowers. Flora was also a "Lady of Pleasure" who delighted in the nude dancing and orgiastic behavior (a wilder version of dancing 'round the Maypole) that took place during her festival. She was so central to Roman religion that her name was said to be the secret soul name of Rome itself. Given the hedonistic lifestyle and unprecedented passion for fragrance among the Romans, it seems quite appropriate. (For a more extensive description of the Romans' use and love of scent, see "Romance of the Rose," chapter 3.)

Erotic aromatherapy borrows from the love practices of many ancient cultures as well as traditions of perfumery and modern scientific and empirical research. Books such as the *Kama Sutra* and *Ananga Ranga* of India, the Tantric scriptures, and the Arab/Islamic *Perfumed Garden* describe sensual practices and erotic wisdom distilled from thousands of years of human experience. Unlike the ascetic Christian tradition popularized by the evangelist Paul just after the turn of the millennium, in which spirituality and sex can have nothing to do with one another, Eastern religious traditions such as Islam, Tantra, Hinduism, and certain sects of Buddhism and Christian Gnosticism continued to embrace the expression of sensuality as an acceptable path to experience the divine. Solomon's two-thousand-year-old love poem the Song of Songs is drenched in scented, erotic imagery:

> While the king was on his couch,
> My nard gave forth its fragrance.
> My beloved to me is a bag of myrrh
> Lodged between my breasts.
> My beloved to me is a spray of henna blooms
> From the vineyards of En-gedi.
>
> Awake, O north wind,
> Come, O south wind!
> Blow upon my garden,
> That its perfume may spread.
>
> Let my beloved come to his garden
> And enjoy its luscious fruits!

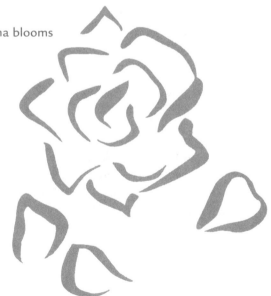

Henna blooms, or camphire, were widely used in the ancient world in perfumes and cosmetics. Cleopatra scented the sails of her barge with camphire for her first meeting with Antony. Muhammad, founder of Islam, who loved both fragrances and the women who wore them, favored the intoxicating aroma of the henna bloom above that of any other flower. The woman's "garden," of course, is an ancient metaphor for the *yoni*, or female sex organ. (*Yoni is* a Sanskrit word meaning sacred space. The male equivalent is the *lingam*, or rod of light.)

In *The Perfumed Garden* a story is recounted of the false Arabian prophet Mocailama, who is challenged to a showdown of divine power by a rival prophetess. One of his followers, a "superior" man, gives the prophet some "father to son" advice. Mocailama is instructed to erect a colorful tent of silk and brocade and to fill it with perfumes of amber, musk, rose, orange flowers, and jasmine, among others. When the aromas have thoroughly permeated the tent, he is to bring in the prophetess, who, he is assured, will become so aroused and disoriented by the fragrances that she will lose all control and submit to his sexual advances. The prophet follows the instructions, and the plan comes off as promised. After the seduction, the prophetess asks to be made his wife, having had "the revelation of God descend" upon her. "The use of perfumes," the book warns, "by man as well as by woman, excites to the act of copulation."

Modern advertisers may not say it so blatantly, but isn't this what designer fragrance billboards and commercials are about? Drive down any busy street, turn on the TV, or open a magazine, and you will see beautiful, half-naked men and women draped over furniture or wrapped around each other. You may or may not notice the little glass bottle that appears in the corner of the ad. Yet the association is powerful, subliminal, and very clear, particularly when the image is accompanied by a fragrance sample to scratch and sniff!

Like *The Perfumed Garden*, Tantric practices incorporate the use of scent in anointing and sensual massage, and the *Kama Sutra* is full of fragrant love potions. Many of the flowers and fragrances suggested by these texts for amorous applications are difficut to find outside their countries of origin, but some are readily available today, and in the following chapters, we will explore them more deeply.

We are indeed fortunate to live during a time when so many rare and precious essences are within relatively easy reach. Using pure, distilled essential oils and floral absolutes, you can re-create for yourself and your lover the atmosphere of Mocailama's tent or a Tantric temple, utilizing aromas that have been prized throughout history by high priests and priestesses, kings, queens, and courtesans, for their aphrodisiac effects.

In the uppermost chamber of the seventh and highest tier of the great tower of Babylon, a perfumed woman was said to recline on a couch, awaiting the amorous pleasure of the Babylonian god Baal when he chose to come down from the higher realms. Was the woman perfumed only to attract Baal's attention? Or were the scents she was anointed with chosen to have a soothing and arousing effect on her as well? What is the nature of the ties that so inextricably bind fragrance to sexual attraction and response?

In another part of Baal's tower stood an enormous statue of the god, cast from pure gold. Before it, on a golden altar, was a perpetually burning brazier filled with frankincense. Why has frankincense, still burned in the Catholic church today, been used as a part of worship for so many thousands of years? Is there a similarity between fragrances used for sensual and religious purposes? How does an aroma alter states of consciousness and mind?

The answers to these questions, and more, lie deep within the human brain, in the structures of the limbic system. But first, let's take a moment to explore how fragrance is perceived.

Smell Perception, or Why There Are No Perfumes in Outer Space

WITHOUT AIR, THERE CAN BE NO SENSE OF SMELL. An aroma is actually composed of bunches of fragrant molecules riding in on the air we breathe. The sensitivity of our olfactory apparatus is truly amazing. We can pick up on and recognize an aroma when odor molecules are present in concentrations as low as a few minuscule parts per million. We are influenced by scents in our environment that are well below the threshold of conscious evaluation. Our bodies and emotions are cued to respond to traces of odors so negligible, we don't even realize they're there.

Each and every human being has a unique aroma, a "smell print" as individual as a fingerprint, though not as static. A fingerprint is a reliable tool for identification because its pattern is unchanging over the course of a lifetime. A smell print, however, is a pattern in a constant state of flux, determined by a variety of factors including genetic makeup, skin type, mood, state of health, what we eat, medicines we take, even the weather! This smell print determines much of our instinctive response to each other, whom we are attracted to, whom we dislike, and with whom we choose to mate or bond.

Contained in the smell print are volumes of information that ride in on the air as we come within smelling distance of each other. The miraculous computer of our brain senses, encodes, and interprets the data within moments of receiving it. We don't get a printout, only a general message conveyed through the body as an emotional or intuitive impression, such as "I like this guy!" "Something's wrong," or "You really turn me on!" (There's even an expression in German, "Ich kann ihn nicht riechen," meaning " I can't smell him," which is a statement of intense dislike.)

A woman's sense of smell is generally more discerning than that of a male, which may provide a biochemical explanation for "women's intuition" and the female's greater sensitivity to the emotional cues and states of others. At the time of ovulation, a woman gives off a scent that a man finds highly appealing and that stimulates him in turn to produce an odor that has an aphrodisiac effect on the woman. Apocrine glands located on the face, around the nipples and navel, under the arms (except among certain Asian people), and in the genital and anal areas of both sexes are believed to release a particular aroma during arousal that indicates sexual readiness. We don't guess at a state of mutual attraction, we literally smell it.

As aroma-rich air flows through the nasal passages, it travels over the olfactory epithelium, tickling tiny filaments (cilia) that protrude from olfactory knobs that form the tips of nerve cells. Each of these cilia is genetically programmed to recognize certain odor molecules, and when they do, they grab on in a kind of welcoming hug. The hug produces a chemical messenger that shoots back along the knob to the olfactory nerve, connected by a direct pathway to the limbic system, cortex, and other areas of the brain. This initiates a rush of electrical activity that forms a pattern, which the brain then organizes, interprets, and ultimately recognizes as a particular smell.

When men and women meet, pheromones are also being mutually sampled and analyzed through the vomeronasal organ, which operates separately from the olfactory system. Pheromones (derived from the Greek words *pherein*, to bear along, and *hormon*, an excitement) are exuded from the skin, secreted with sweat. They relay messages that contribute to sexual arousal in the opposite sex, as well as communicate negative states of being such as anxiety or fear.

In the time it takes to shake hands, two strangers have already made sensory decisions about each other that will determine whether or not they choose to commit themselves to the process of "olfactory bonding," now recognized by scientists as the glue that holds deep human relationships together, including family ties, friendships, and romantic alliances.

To illustrate the importance of olfactory function to sexuality, animals and people born lacking a sense of smell tend to have sexual dysfunctions as well, such as underdeveloped reproductive organs and lack of sexual response. Those who lose their sense of smell in the course of life also suffer from diminished libido and hormonal disturbances.

The Limbic System: "Pleasure Central"

THE INTENSE ASSOCIATIONS BETWEEN EMOTIONS, sexual response, memory, and the sense of smell can be explained by the fact that the olfactory system is the only one of our senses that projects directly into the brain via the limbic system. Located deep within the brain, the limbic system is a complex of structures that mediates between the ancient, reptilian brain's preoccupation with survival and the computerlike, problem-solving higher functions of the cerebral cortex. The limbic system is the seat of our emotions, imagination, playfulness, maternal instinct, and basic drives and is tightly interconnected with the hypothalamus, which controls hormonal levels and sexual rhythms. It is also directly linked to the hippocampus, one of the earliest developed parts of the brain, which is involved in the processing of sensory input. The amygdala, part of the limbic system, together with the hippocampus, orchestrates memory.

Unlike other senses, such as vision, which must travel via more convoluted neural pathways, olfactory fibers have direct contact with the hippocampus and amygdala, which explains the inordinate power of smells to trigger cascades of remembered events. Fragrances become associated with loved ones, happy times, and youthful experiences. Many writers have commented on the ability of a sudden whiff of a cherished aroma to transport us unexpectedly, instantaneously, into vivid memories of another time and place. Often these memory transports are accompanied by overwhelming, almost aching rushes of feeling. In a study sposored by the Fragrance Research fund, the powerful link between fragrance and memory is demonstrated. People have been shown to recall smells with 65% accuracy after a year has elapsed, whereas estimated visual recall of photographs was shown to be a low 50% after only three months.

Through the hypothalmus and the limbic system run the pathways that create our perception of pleasure. How important is pleasure to our existence? The behavior of all animals, human beings included, is driven on a basic level by the desire to experience pleasure or to avoid pain. Feelings of pleasure are accompanied by intense electrical activity in the limbic structures of the brain, which is why I refer to it as "Pleasure Central." Test animals with electrodes planted in these areas of their brains, given the ability to create pleasurable sensations by depressing a lever, chose pleasure over food, water, sleep, and all other activities. They did nothing all day long but depress the levers! Compassionate scientists eventually unhooked the poor things before they starved to death.

Because of the olfactory system's direct wiring into Pleasure Central, our reaction to an odor is immediate, primitive, visceral, and intense, causing an instantaneous and measurable rise in our level of physiological arousal. We are thinking creatures, and (theoretically) able to derail our instinctive responses at will. Still, it's difficult to ignore our sense of smell and the information it conveys. We can close our eyes and mouths, stop up our ears, back off from an embrace, but we can't stop breathing. Olfactory information stimulates us constantly and relentlessly, whether or not we choose to act on the state of arousal it creates.

The Smell of Love and the Point of Perfume

IN PERFUMERY, especially as the art has been perfected over the centuries in France, chemical constituents of certain fragrant essences and absolutes are recognized as having the capacity to produce particular effects on mood and psyche. A good perfume is not just a pretty smell; it is meant to create an erotic sensation. For the French, a perfume without aphrodisiac properties is like a car with no gas. If it's not going anywhere, what's the point?

Perfume materials and fragrance compounds are categorized according to whether their effects are erogenic (inducing erotic feelings), antierogenic, stimulating, or narcotic. Narcotic aromas have an effect similar to any other narcotic substance, tending to reduce the dominance of the rational and logical mind, thereby opening the gate to the subconscious and releasing the conditioned, "civilized" hold on primitive impulses. A narcotic effect, however, is not by nature erotic; it simply releases inhibition and heightens the senses. Incense with narcotic aromatic elements is often burned during religious ceremonies to open the worshiper to an experience of spiritual ecstasy. The same aromatic substance, used in different surroundings, might act as an aphrodisiac.

Rose is a good example of this. Long associated with both spiritual and sensual love, the aroma of rose owes its intoxicating reputation to the presence of certain narcotic alcohols. Yet the fragrance of rose, in and of itself, is not necessarily erotic. In order for an aroma to work as an aphrodisiac, it must also include aromatic elements that are sexually provocative and elements that are stimulating and refreshing. Rose is the most beloved fragrance in the world and an important element in perfume blending, having been used in 42% of masculine fragrances, and 96% of women's perfumes up until the 1980s (*The H&R Book of Perfume*). But based on fragrance composition alone, jasmine is the sexier essence, containing elements that simultaneously cause relaxation and arousal, the combination necessary to pitch awareness into an erotic state.

This is just what happened to Mocailama's prophetess. She didn't stand a chance once she entered his tent! Everything around her was impregnated with aphrodisiac perfumes. Every breath she took was loaded with seductive aromatic innuendo. Narcotic components of rose and neroli went to work first, relaxing her body, subduing her critical faculties, and opening the gates of the senses, which were further stimulated by the sensual colors and textures of silk furniture and hanging brocades. Mocailama, making sure he was alone with her, "engaged her in conversation," which enabled him to witness the weakening of her rational thought processes while simultaneously fixing her attention on himself. Amorous fantasies engendered by the erogenic qualities of the flower perfumes were then focused in his direction, while the frank sexual messages of aromatic substances like musk and amber took care of the rest.

It's interesting to note that no truly aphrodisiac perfume can be formulated without a few aromatic elements that resemble sweat, feces, and decay. The most striking of these naturally occurring elements is indole, which is present in the perfumes of all the delicate, white, moth-pollinated blossoms known for their aphrodisiac aromas, such as jasmine, narcissus, madonna lily, tuberose, and lilac. Indole is closely related chemically to scatol, which is the active component in civet, a foul-smelling excretion from the sex glands of an untamable mammal of the same name. (Diluted to infinitesimal levels, civet has a pleasant floral fragrance that is integral to many perfumes.) Indole is also a part of the inimitable odor of putrefaction, the rotting of flesh. So why do we register it as "sexy"? While we're being transported by delightful aromas that plants and flowers have created from springtime and sunlight, we need to be reminded, it seems, ever so fleetingly, of our mortality and our animal nature. Desire is heightened by a subtle reminder of the ancient Greek idea that Love is a sudden and inexplicable radiance born from darkness and Death, and we should enjoy it while we can!

The "Big O," or Love, Orgasm, and Oxytocin

ORGASM (from the Greek *orgasmos*, to swell with wetness) is one of those wonderful mysteries that we all know about but can't fully explain. For all our technology, we know amazingly little about ourselves. We surmise that orgasmic capacity, on an emotional and psychological level, requires a healthy ability to let go occasionally, to allow emotion and feeling to eclipse thought, to permit the id a kind of holiday, a moment of transcendence over the ego. Spiritually, orgasm opens us to an experience of fusion and oneness with what we normally perceive to be "outside" ourselves: our lover, and the all-encompassing flow of surrounding reality.

On a physical level, the climax of lovemaking is stimulated by a combination of touch, movement, breath, and the gradual build up of a hormone called oxytocin, which is thought to trigger the rapid firing of genital nerves resulting in a sudden, overwhelming flood of feeling and sensation. Levels of this "pleasure hormone" are five times higher than normal in men during orgasm. Women require even more oxytocin to reach climax, and their oxytocin levels exceed those of men during arousal. The same hormone, incidentally, brings on labor, stimulates contractions during and after childbirth, and causes the letdown reflex in a nursing mother, when milk flows in response to the sound of her baby's hungry cries. For a woman, the pleasures of maternal and sexual response flow along the same neural pathways. Cuddling with a loved one, nurturing a child at the breast, giving birth, and reaching sexual climax are all, at a biochemical level, similar in feeling to women. This may explain such things as the orgasm some women report experiencing during childbirth, the sexual arousal some mothers feel during nursing, and women's increased orgasmic capacity following the birth of a child. While men's oxytocin levels also rise during cuddling and sex, and in response to their children, the pitch is less steep.

Oxytocin response can be conditioned by smells and fragrances associated with a lover, as well as by the body processes described above. You can literally condition an arousal response through the use of aromas that become associated with the excitement of intimacy and the warm feelings that you and your partner share. The aromatherapy blend you use on a regular basis with your lover thus becomes a key that can unlock an automatic pleasure response.

Now that we have a sense of why aromatherapy for lovers is so powerful and effective, let's explore some of the essences of love.

TWO

The Essences of Love

How to Use Essential Oils

THE POSSIBILITIES ARE ENDLESS, limited only by the boundaries of your romantic imagination. Essential oils can be diffused into the air and breathed in, dropped into a bath to soak in, splashed on in the form of waters or colognes, and used in perfume or massage oils to penetrate the skin. **Caution: Do not drink any mixture containing essential oils described in this book!** Essential oils taken internally can have a damaging effect on the liver and internal organs, and should never be ingested without the guidance of a qualified physician. When using an essence or carrier you haven't tried before, be sure to spot test a small amount on the inside of your arm (or your lover's) to check yourselves for any possible sensitivity to the substance before using it over a larger area.

Aromatherapy for lovers, like practical aromatherapy, uses pure essential oils that are distilled from plant materials such as flowers, stems, leaves, seeds, and roots.

Because many of Nature's most seductive aromas are too delicate to survive the heat of the distillation process that produces the most commonly used essential oils, aromatherapy for lovers also includes the use of floral absolutes such as jasmine and tuberose, which are won by less intense processes, such as solvent extraction or enfleurage. (See Chapter 8 for a description of distillation methods.)

The difference between aromatherapy for lovers and the use of perfume or over-the-counter products is, first, the assurance that you're using a high-quality, naturally derived fragrant material and, second, that you are the creator of your own experience, choosing with conscious intention the erotic effect you want most to inspire, in the most beautifully aromatic way you know how!

To avoid disappointment and ensure the greatest possible success with your blends, I encourage you to buy the best-quality oils you can find. By doing so, you not only train your nose and aesthetic sense to the highest level of refinement, you encourage and ensure the continued availability of fine aromatic essences and absolutes.

The finest aphrodisiac essences do not come cheap. If they do, they're either very low grade or synthetics masquerading as genuine oils. Be prepared to pay for rare and costly essences such as rose, jasmine, iris, tuberose, narcissus, neroli, and melissa. Midrange aphrodisiac essences include ylang-ylang, patchouli, lavender, vetiver, geranium, and spice oils. Again, you can find lower grades for less money, and you can find rare varieties of usually low- or midrange oils that command a high price. Citrus essences tend to be at the lower end of the price spectrum because of their greater availability.

Aromatic diffusers can be as simple as five-dollar ceramic rings that fit over your light bulb or as complex as the professional electric models that pump air through a system of glass baffles and turn the essence into a fine mist sprayed throughout a room. Potpourri burners can also be used, and there are some beautiful candle-warmed burners created just for essential oil use available from companies listed at the end of this book. Essential oils, individually or in blends, should be used neat, or undiluted, in diffusers. Use alcohol to clean out your diffuser between blends, especially after viscous or sticky essences such as sandalwood or vetiver have been used.

Aromatherapy candles can be purchased or made at home from kits available at craft stores. Essential oils are added when the wax is liquid and starting to cool. You can also add a few drops to an unscented candle after lighting it by placing the essence in the liquid pool of wax that collects around the wick as the candle burns.

Reserve your best essences for baths, massage oils, and perfumes, however. When you've invested in a precious essence, you don't want to waste a molecule! Because essential oils are attracted to the fats in your skin, they get right down to business when externally applied. Twenty minutes in a warm tub should ensure that you've absorbed or inhaled all the essence. After receiving an aromatherapy massage, be sure to wait at least an hour before showering or bathing to allow time for the blend to be absorbed completely.

The essences recommended in the book, if purchased from reliable aromatherapy essential oil suppliers, should be quite safe for you to use. Additional safety information is included in the charts at the end of this book.

Getting to Know Your Essential Oils

ESSENTIAL OILS HAVE UNIQUE PERSONALITIES, and each year's distillation will differ slightly in aroma and chemical composition. The labor and time required to grow and process plants for their essential oils are only two of the reasons the essences are relatively expensive, especially when compared to synthetic perfume fragrances that can be mass-produced in laboratories out of petrochemical by-products. Most essential oil crops are grown or wild-crafted by small producers who live close to the land. Essential oil-bearing plants will often thrive and produce a superior grade of essence only in a certain climate zone in a particular geographic area. The plants are highly vulnerable to changing weather conditions; too much rain or an unexpected drought can ruin a crop, and with it the availability of an essential oil for that year.

Certain oils, such as the citruses, are less expensive and more readily available because the fruits that produce them are widely cultivated for juice and produce. Other plants, such as helichrysm, are grown only for their essential oils, in very remote, specific locations by a handful of dedicated growers, and thus are rare and costly.

Another factor determining cost is how much plant material it takes to produce the essential oil. Herbaceous materials such as marjoram and rosemary contain considerably more essence than do most of the florals, such as jasmine or rose. Essence of sandalwood is not even produced in the tree until it has reached at least twenty-five years of age.

If you really want to understand essential oils, you'll have to take time to get to know them, as you would any new acquaintance. You won't know all about an oil no matter how much you read about its properties, chemical composition, and traditional uses. The most intimate knowledge will come from your own personal experiences.

Pick just a few essences to start with; spend some time with them. Breathe in the aromatic vapor of the essence from its open bottle or vial. How does it make you feel? Put a tiny drop on your skin, and notice how the fragrance changes. Does it feel good on your skin? Does it itch or tingle? Note any intuitive response you have to the essence: Where do you respond to it in your body? Some oils feel as if they get stuck in your throat; others seem to penetrate down to the soles of your feet. Try to verbalize the message the aroma seems to be giving you.

Essential oils are a bridge between the world of humans and the world of plants. Each time you use an essence with love, awareness, and appreciation, you strengthen the web that connects all life on Earth. The more honor and respect you accord your oils, the better your blends will be, in both form and function. Try it and see!

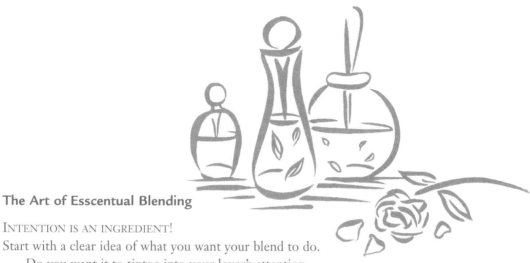

The Art of Esscentual Blending

INTENTION IS AN INGREDIENT!
Start with a clear idea of what you want your blend to do.

Do you want it to tiptoe into your lover's attention, all soft and sweet? Or is a sudden and passionate conflagration more what you have in mind? Choose a few essences whose aromas and properties seem to fit your intention, then sit down in a quiet, fragrance-free room with plenty of time to play and a notebook and pencil to record what you've done.

The best way to blend is to put your essential oils together first, before adding the carrier. This allows optimal contact among molecules of the various oils to create a strong synergy in which the effect of the whole is often greater than the sum of the parts. Until you're experienced with the various aromas, however, the fragrance of pure essences may be too intense for you to get a clear picture of how it's going to smell in dilution.

So start with the second-best way. Add the essences, a drop or two at a time, to a bottle half full of carrier, such as sweet almond or safflower oil. Go slowly, and sniff after each addition, gently swishing the bottle to mix. This is a sensual experience: take your time. It's amazing what a difference a single drop of oil can make in a blend. When the smell in the bottle matches the intention created in your mind, try a little bit of the blend on your skin. It may smell completely different. It will also have a different smell on your skin than on someone else's. The most volatile oils, or "top notes," will impress your nose first; these are usually light and fleeting essences that evaporate quickly, such as tangerine and bergamot. They serve to get your attention, and to mask odors in the environment. "Middle notes," such as lavender, evaporate next. The "base notes" are the heavier-smelling, more viscous oils, such as sandalwood, vanilla, and clary sage, and will linger longest on the skin.

The word "esscentual" describes the deliberate use of fragrant essential oils for the purpose of enhancing and awakening sensual experience and desire, and following are some esscentual fragrance "chords" to get you started with blending. These are groups of three to four amorous essences that go well together and should result in a sexy fragrance no matter how you blend them. When you feel more confident, go on to intermediate blending, and improvise by choosing from the complete list of love essences.

Fragrance Chords

Geranium	Ylang-ylang	Neroli	Nutmeg
Lavender	Patchouli	Petitgrain	Vanilla
Clove	Orange	Tangerine	Sandalwood
Jasmine	Clary Sage	Lime	Rose
Bergamot	Chamomile	Bay laurel	Frankincense
Sandalwood	Coriander	Lavender	Benzoin
Black pepper	Cedar		

Base Notes

Ambrette	Bay laurel	Benzoin	Cedarwood
Clary sage	Cistus	Costus	Frankincense
Myrrh	Oakmoss	Patchouli	Peru balsam
Tolu balsam	Tonka bean	Vanilla	Vetiver

Middle Notes

Basil	Black pepper	Chamomile	Fennel
Geranium	Ginger	Lavender	Marjoram
Myrtle	Nutmeg	Palmarosa	Pine
Rosemary	Rosewood	Ylang-ylang	

Top Notes

All citruses	Angelica	Bergamot	Cardamom
Cinnamon	Clove	Coriander	Hyacinth
Iris	Juniper	Melissa	Neroli
Peppermint	Petitgraine		

Multinote

MIDDLE/BASE

Jasmine	Ylang-ylang	Tuberose	Narcissus

MIDDLE/TOP

Carnation	Champac	Rose

Extenders

(use up to 50% to extend precious essences)

Geranium (with rose)	Lavender	Orange
Palmarosa (with rose)	Rosewood	Tangerine

Binders

(help to hold a blend together)

Benzoin   Lavender   Rosewood   Vanilla

Recommended Dilutions

BATHS: Use **5–15 drops** in a tub, depending on the sensitivity of your skin and the essence you've chosen. Try diluting potentially irritating oils, such as citruses or spice essences, in a tablespoon of milk or cold-pressed nut oil. If you still experience irritation, use less of the essence or try another combination.

MASSAGE OILS: Use **5–10 drops** of essence per ounce of carrier oil, again depending on skin sensitivity and the essence chosen. The fragrance intensity of certain oils, such as ylang-ylang, geranium, and jasmine, is so pronounced that as you blend you'll naturally find yourself using less to get the effect you want. Other essences, such as rosewood and lavender, are nonirritating and have lower fragrance intensity, meaning you can use greater quantities to fill out a blend or for skin-soothing or calming effects.

PERFUMES: Because you apply only a drop or two at a time, perfume blends can be highly concentrated, using as much as 100 drops per half ounce of a stable carrier such as jojoba oil. Be careful of dermal irritation, and dilute or change your blend if you have a reaction to it.

Carrier Oils

YOU CAN MIX YOUR FAVORITE ESSENTIAL OILS into unscented, commercially available shampoos, creams, or shower gels. You can also create your own perfume, bath, and massage goodies using oils, vinegars, or alcohol as carriers. There are recipes sprinkled throughout the book, and additional ones in the last chapter. But making up your own blends is the most fun. Any of the following oils are nourishing to the skin and good to use for bath, body, and massage oil blends, provided you get an oil that has been cold or expeller pressed and is thus solvent-free. Low grades of oils are sometimes created by wringing out the last oily dregs of previous expeller pressings with chemical solvents such as hexane. Such oils are not appropriate for aromatherapeutic use.

SWEET ALMOND OIL: A love goddess oil. The almond has long been a symbol of the female *yoni*, and was said to have sprung from the genitals of the ancient Phrygian fertility goddess Cybele, who was worshiped in Greece, Rome, and throughout the Near East from 6000 B.C. to about the 4th century A.D. Previously easy to find, a recent lowering of standards for whole almonds has resulted in fewer of the nuts being pressed into oil. Stable, nutritious, and easily absorbed into the skin.

APRICOT KERNEL OIL: Light and nourishing, not as stable as sweet almond.

AVOCADO OIL: Heavy, rich oil, great for dry, dehydrated skin.

BORAGE SEED OIL: Comprised of up to one-fourth gamma linoleic acid (GLA), which reinforces the skin and improves its function as a protective membrane. Use up to 10% in your blend to heal and regenerate skin.

CANOLA OIL: Also known as rapeseed oil, light and quick to absorb.

CARROT SEED OIL: Actually an essential oil, a few drops in a blend will add vitamins, minerals, and beta carotene. Try adding it to a moisturizing facial oil made of $1/2$ ounce hazelnut oil, 20 drops of rosa mosqueta, and a few drops of rose.

EVENING PRIMROSE OIL: Another GLA-rich oil, rejuvenating to the skin and useful for balancing underlying physiological functions.

GRAPESEED OIL: Very light and quick to absorb.

HAZELNUT OIL: My favorite! Rich, nourishing, great for skin care.

JOJOBA OIL: Not really an oil, but a wax, and a perfect base for perfume oils because it doesn't become rancid. A good hair-conditioning oil. Add a few drops to a facial oil blend to increase emollience.

OLIVE OIL: A bit sticky and strong smelling, but good for hair and skin care.

PEANUT OIL: Good basic oil, easy to find.

PECAN OIL: Light, stable, nourishing.

ROSEHIP SEED OIL: Also known as *rosa mosqueta* and *rosa rubignosa*, this GLA-rich oil has properties similar to evening primrose oil. Also good for facial and skin care. Nutritious, emollient, and regenerative.

SAFFLOWER OIL: Good basic massage oil for all skin types.

SESAME OIL: A great oil for men. In India, sesame is known as a *rasayana*, or life extender, and is esteemed in all its forms as a virility food. Light, nourishing, and warming, with a high content of vitamin E. As of this writing, it's also very hard to find because of recent crop failures. Unrefined oil will make you smell like a stir fry. Stick with refined.

SUNFLOWER OIL: Good basic oil.

WHEATGERM OIL: Very rich, high vitamin E content, which makes it a good oil to blend with other oils for its antioxidant effects (helps prevent rancidity).

VITAMIN E: Nourishing skin support. Squeeze in one capsule per ounce of carrier oil as a natural preservative.

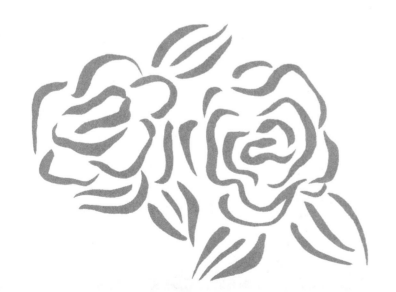

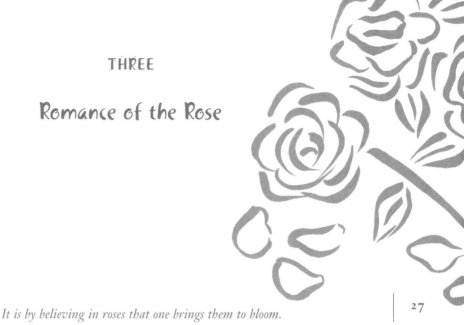

THREE

Romance of the Rose

It is by believing in roses that one brings them to bloom.
FRENCH PROVERB

THE ROSE IS SACRED TO LOVERS AND MYSTICS. To the Sufis, mystics of Islamic tradition, its elegant bloom atop a dense, thorned cane epitomizes the path to God. Likewise the rose represents the arduous journey of true lovers, whose thorny struggles toward intimacy are ultimately rewarded by an unfolding of love's grace and beauty, the blossoming of the heart.

Use essence of rose at the beginning of a love relationship to ease gently the fears that accompany opening the heart, fears that can resurface at any stage of intimacy. Rose is the perfect choice for those who have been scarred on love's battlefield and who may have difficulty surrendering themselves unreservedly to love's rosy glow. If this description fits you or your lover, take it easy, take it slow, and indulge each other with a tender rub using the Rose Petal Caress massage blend included in your kit.

Stroke a teaspoon of the oil over the area of the heart, where rose's sweet reassurance can soften and penetrate the most rigid armor. Heart massage with rose not only opens the way for new connections but also helps to reestablish intimacy damaged by a misunderstanding or lovers' spat.

Whereas the delicate, ephemeral fragrances of honeysuckle, violet, and hyacinth are akin to flirtations of the flower world, pleasing but short-lived and difficult to retain, rose is a deep and enduring devotion. One of the few flowers able to withstand the heat of the distillation process without a loss or destruction of scent, rose perseveres, as does true love, withstanding the ravages of time and experience with its sweetness left intact.

Aromatherapy and the Rose

MODERN AROMATHERAPEUTIC USES FOR ROSE OIL and rose water parallel those recorded since ancient times by physicians and historians. Because the chemistry of rose water is virtually identical to that of rose essential oil, genuine rose water can be thought of as a dilute form of rose oil. This dilute form may be more appropriate for the very young, the elderly, and those with extremely sensitive constitutions. It is also excellent for the treatment of subtle problems, such as anxiety, lack of confidence, and emotional turmoil. The 16th-century *Grete Herbal* suggested rose water be taken internally by "them that be faynt at the herte." (And what lover isn't, from time to time?) Jan Salko, who imports Bulgarian rose essence and rose water, confirms this application, as do many other modern-day aromatherapists. Rosewater can be found in Middle Eastern specialty food stores and in some liquor stores, or by contacting Jan's company, "Sensory Essence" (see the resource guide at the back of the book).

Rose water was used by the ancient Romans to combat the effects of overindulgence in food and wine. The Arab physician Ibn Sina was using attar of roses for ailments of the digestive tract over a thousand years ago, and modern research confirms its efficacy. A study published in 1988 indicates rose water's "prophylactic and therapeutic properties in gastrointestinal, renal, and liver diseases."

Rose essence is the most antiseptic of all the flower oils, having seven times more germicidal strength than carbolic acid. Recent research done in Bulgaria, such as that presented at the 1994 Bulgarian Rose Conference by Dr. Raicho Tse Vetkov Raev, Head of the Institute for Roses, Essential Oil, and Medicinal Plants, confirms the antibacterial properties of rose water. Research done by Kirov & Vankov published in *Medica-Biologic Information* in 1988, shows rose water to be effective against streptococci, staphylococci, diptheria bacteria, anthrax bacillus, and coli. Ayurvedic practitioners have traditionally used rose petals in poultices to treat skin wounds and inflammations.

Rose water has been used worldwide to treat eye inflammations and diseases such as conjunctivitis. Taken internally in small amounts, it is said to strengthen the heart. Bulgarian research points to a multitude of applications, from eye, mouth, and skin conditions to feminine hygiene and the treatment of diarrhea. Rose has additionally been shown to balance bile production in the liver and to assist in decholesterolization of the blood.

In the practice of aromatherapy, rose is used sparingly because of its high cost and relative unavailability. It can be very difficult to find an essence that is authentic and pure enough for aromatherapeutic use. This is a shame, because of rose's wide range of potentially beneficial applications.

Robert Tisserand found rose beneficial in the treatment of heart problems and blood circulation. On a subtle level, rose opens the heart, soothing such heart-constricting problems as anger, fear, anxiety, disharmony, and depression.

A 1:2 ratio of rose to melissa oil is mentioned by the German chemist Dietrich

Wabner as effective in the treatment of herpes zoster and herpes simplex. The oil is applied undiluted two or three times a day. Equal amounts of melissa (essence of lemon balm) and rose oil diluted in jojoba oil, applied to the temples, fights headaches and migraines. (Genuine melissa, however, can be even more difficult to find than rose.) Wabner also recommends 30 drops of rose oil in 10 ml (one-third ounce) of jojoba for bruises and a 10:1 blend of lavender to rose for bruises and wounds.

Rose is a wonderful overall tonic to invigorate and strengthen the body and to increase emotional balance and equanimity on all levels of being. It has also been known for thousands of years as a potent aphrodisiac. Bulgarian women have a saying: "Put rose water in his thermos and he'll be home on time for dinner."

Cleopatra was well acquainted with the aphrodisiacal properties of rose. To impress Antony on his first visit, she greeted him from atop an eighteen-inch-deep carpet of rose petals, held in place by nets fastened to the walls. At one of his orgies, the lascivious emperor Nero asphyxiated a guest with a shower of rose petals that fell from his ceiling. A friend of Nero's once spent the equivalent of $100,000 on roses for a single dinner party.

Because its affinity to the female reproductive system is unparalleled by any other essential oil, rose is used extensively for these purposes. Marguerite Maury, noting the wide use of rose oil among the Hindus, found it to have a purifying and regulating effect on the female sexual organs. Since ancient times, when it was sacred to Aphrodite, rose has always held a special place in the hearts, minds, and bodies of women.

Greek, Roman, and Egyptian women used roses in perfume and bathed their faces in rose water to preserve the beauty and softness of their skin, a practice still recommended today by the French herbalist Maurice Messegue, among others.

In the arid deserts of the Middle East, rose water was drunk as a cooling, healthful beverage and incorporated into sherbets, pastries, and other culinary delicacies. Guests were welcomed with a sprinkle of rose water from a special vessel known as a *gulabdan.* (As modern research attests to the antiseptic power of rose, it occurs to me that this may have been the subtle equivalent of spraying incoming visitors with Lysol.)

The wide diversity of aromatherapeutic applications for essence of rose and rose water is explained by the extreme chemical complexity of the oil. The most complex of all essential oils, genuine rose contains more than 300 chemical constituents. Almost 200 of these are not yet identified and are found in trace amounts in less than 2% of the oil. Despite their minuscule amounts, these traces play an important part in the fullness and beauty of rose's unique fragrance.

Rose essence won from the Damask rose of the Kazanlik Valley in Bulgaria is chemically characterized by a predominance of free alcohols, the most abundant of which is citronellol, known for its antirheumatic and insecticide effects. Other dominant compounds include geraniol, nerol, phenyl-ethanol, which are anesthetic and bacteriostatic, and farnesol, another bactericide that is also beneficial to the skin and mucous membranes. Farnesol, which also occurs in a number of other essential oils, retards staphylococcus and functions as a natural, skin-friendly deodorant. Dehydroisoionone, a trace component at $1/10$ of a percent, is what gives a Damask rose its characteristic fragrance.

French Centifolia rose contains the same components, but in very different proportions. In the French absolute, the dominant compound is phenyl-ethanol, at more than 60%.

Despite its strength, rose is a gentle giant of aromatherapy, having the least toxic properties of any essential oil. A pure, authentic essence of rose surpasses even a good lavender in terms of mildness and benefit to the skin.

Roses, Old and New

ROSE LOVERS SEPARATE GARDEN ROSES into two very different groups: "old roses" and "modern roses." Old roses are considered to be those introduced before the first hybrid tea rose "La France" in the year 1867. Modern roses, according to the American Rose Society, were introduced after that date. Hybrid tea roses have so dominated the garden scene in the last hundred years that they have come to define our mental picture of the "perfect" rose: a big, half-opened bud of red, yellow, or white crowning the end of a long and graceful stem.

The natural and original color of roses, however, is pink, which is, coincidentally, the vibrational color of love in metaphysical circles. The single blossoms, long stems, and multitude of colors available in modern roses are the results of hybridization.

Essential oils, ottos, and absolutes of rose used in aromatherapy are obtained exclusively from old rose species.

The earliest known depiction of a rose is part of a 4,000-year-old fresco on a wall of the Palace of Minos, in Knossos, Crete. The rose represented there is similar to the Damask rose still cultivated today in Bulgaria. A variety of Damask rose has also been unearthed, still fragrant, in Egyptian tombs. This is the rose that was preserved through the centuries in monastic gardens, and the beloved flower of Islam and the Sufi poets. When Muhammad declared "Whosoever would smell my scent would smell the rose," he was talking about *Rosa damascena*.

The Kazanlik rose, *R. damascena trigentipetala*, was brought by the Turks to Bulgaria, where it is still cultivated for its oil today. The Kazanlik Valley runs across Bulgaria from east to west, protected from weather extremes by hills to the north and south. About 7,000 rose plants will grow on an acre of ground. Two thousand rose blossoms will produce about 2 grams of essential oil. The blossoms are hand-picked at sunrise while the petals are still dewy, during the months of May and early June, and placed in baskets and sacks. The petals are submerged in water, which is then heated, the essence being carried away on the resulting steam and separated by cooling. Double, even triple distillation is sometimes necessary to separate out the essence, due to rose oil's solubility in water. This, and the intensive labor, is what makes rose essence so expensive.

The rose fields are propagated from cuttings of healthy plants and will produce oil for ten to forty years if properly tended. From these fields comes most of the rose essence produced in the world. "Rose bulgare" and Bulgarian rose water are generally agreed to be the finest quality available. (This is the rose used in the "Rose Petal Caress" massage blend included in your kit.)

The Alba, another ancient rose brought to Britain by the Romans and grown extensively in the Middle Ages for medicinal purposes, was the result of a natural hybridization between the Damask rose and *R. canina*, the "dog rose." The white Alba rose was grown in Spain as early as the 12th century, along with the red Damask.

R. alba semi-plena is the Bulgarian white rose grown in the Valley of Kazanlik, prized for the beauty and rarity of its fragrance. *R. gallica* is the ancient "red rose" cultivated by the Greeks, Romans, and Egyptians. Also known as the French rose and the rose of Anatolia, it has been grown for centuries in France for distillation of its essence, hence its name. The Romans grew so many of these roses on the Campanian plains that it was humorously suggested that the extensive space devoted to their cultivation might cause a shortage of grain. This is the rose that was adopted as the emblem of the house of Lancaster during the Wars of the Roses. *R. gallica officinalis* is commonly known as the Apothecary's Rose, due to the wide variety of its traditional medicinal applications.

R. centifolia is also distilled for its essence, and was first bred by the Dutch in the 17th century. Also known as rose de mai, it is cultivated in Grasse, in the south of France, where it is harvested after a single blooming period in spring. Since World War II, Morocco has become the largest source for this rose essence, the price of which is considerably less than that of Bulgarian. Gardeners know it as the cabbage rose.

Of the 250 species of rose that grow throughout the Northern Hemisphere, only these four are cultivated on any scale for their fragrant essence and the rose water that is a by-product of the distillation process.

Old roses commemorate ancient origins and associations in their given names. Among varieties of Damask roses, the Belle Isis smells of myrrh, the incense that once fragranced Egyptian temples. Hyppolyte is named for the Queen of the Amazons; Leda for the mother of Helen of Troy; Hebe's Lip for the Greek goddess of youth and wife of Hercules. The Centifolia rose Juno is named for Hebe's mother, the wife of Zeus.

New roses, the ubiquitous hybrid teas, likewise honor the icons of more modern times: Dolly Parton, Elizabeth Taylor, Cary Grant, Bing Crosby, Helmut Schmidt, Christian Dior, and Pelé, to name but a few.

Roses reflect our most cherished dreams and wishes: "Peace," "Love," "Pleasure," "Confidence," "Esperanza" (Hope), "Hermosa" (Beauty). They can take us "Over the Rainbow" to "Paradise" or "Camelot" on a "Fragrant Cloud" of "Perfume Delight," leaving us happily "Bewitched" and in a state of "Sheer Bliss"!

I encourage you to grow roses in containers or beds close to your home, near places you often pass by, where, as the English rose breeder David Austin has so eloquently put it, their beauty and fragrance can provide "one of those small but not insignificant parts of our life that makes it worth the living." The sight and aroma of my rosebushes blooming as I leave in the morning for work or when I return at the end of a particularly grueling day, lightens my heart with an indescribable sprinkling of joy and delight. On really bad (or good!) days, I head straight for the tub with my vial of rose essence. Six to eight drops can completely erase a foul mood, and as little as one or two drops can envelop and uplift the droopiest spirits. Rose has a way of making everything rise to its own level of peace and beauty . . . or is it just that trace narcotic component of its chemistry that makes it seem so?

Plant old roses near a bedroom window that gets the morning sun, and be awakened each morning by a fragrance that has been the very breath of love for thousands of years!

The Rose Meditation

THROUGHOUT A LIFETIME OF OBSERVING MYSELF and those around me, I've come to the conclusion that most of the pain and suffering people feel in their close and intimate relationships is due to a sudden, awful feeling that they're no longer lovable, or no longer loved. Unraveling the causes for this can spark a lifetime search for self-knowledge and understanding. While I encourage that pursuit, I also recommend regular indulgence in the following simple meditation, as both an antidote to and preventive medicine for, feelings of emotional abandonment. The heart-opening aroma of rose helps us to remember that we are all loved deeply, all the time. Use rose whenever you need to remember that love is the bottom line of reality, the distilled essence of who we really are and why we are here.

I AM LOVE. Sit quietly and comfortably, somewhere that you can expect not to be disturbed. Using rose essence or absolute, or the Rose Petal Caress blend from your kit, anoint the area over your heart and also your throat, upper lip, and forehead, if you so desire.

Breathe slowly and deeply. Close your eyes, and focus your energy within. Relax your chest and shoulders, relax your throat, let your tongue float inside your mouth. Let the tension drain out of your neck and face. Let your eyes relax. Sink into the chair, pillow, or floor where you're sitting. Let your whole body relax. Now focus again on the aroma of the rose and the message it has to convey. There is nothing you need to do to be loved. Imagine a place at the center of existence, the beating heart of the universe, the secret dwelling place of a Higher Power. This is where you come from. You are love, precipitated into human form. Meditate on the words "I am love" and what they mean to you. Allow a feeling of love to well up inside you, to radiate from and into every cell in your body.

I AM LOVING. Just as the aromatic essence of rose projects itself through the air to connect so sweetly and lovingly with your senses, you can project rays of affection invisibly to the people you love. Picture a loved one now in your mind. Feel your connection to that person as a ray of love that travels from your heart to theirs. Imagine that you are sprinkling them with the pink and gold dust of your affection. See them glowing and basking in a transparent pink aura created by your positive regard. How many people do you feel that way about? Send love to them; friends, family, those who have helped you, influenced you, or taught you something important along life's way. Try to include them all.

I AM LOVED. Now reverse the flow of energy in the circle of connection you've created with those you love. Let your heart open like a rose to accept the flow of love coming back from them to you. Feel a sense of appreciation and gratitude for their presence in your life, and the emotional and spiritual sustenance you and your loved ones mutually provide. Let thoughts float through and away from you now, as you simply experience the flow of love through your being, allowing its current to carry you effortlessly through these moments of life. When you're ready, take a few deep, closing breaths and open your eyes. Allow the feelings you've experienced to accompany you through the rest of your day.

FOUR

The Esscentual Woman

Her rowers caressed the water with oars of silver, which dipped in time to the music of the flute, accompanied by pipes and lutes . . . Instead of a crew the barge was lined with the most beautiful of her waiting women attired as Nereids [sea nymphs] and Graces, some at the rudders, others at the tackles of the sails, and all the while an indescribably rich perfume, exhaled from innumerable censers, was wafted from the vessel to the river banks.

PLUTARCH, *from eyewitness accounts of Cleopatra's arrival into Tarsus*

Cleopatra

NO WOMAN IS BETTER KNOWN for "scentual" smarts and seductiveness than Cleopatra. Fragrance, allure, and a flair for the dramatic were her birthright as queen of the Egyptian empire. Descended from Alexander the Great through the Ptolemies, she was wealthy beyond imagining, manipulative, intelligent, and politically savvy, and she spoke numerous languages, including Latin, Greek, and the obscure dialects of her own far-flung subjects.

Women in ancient Egypt were honored, educated, and had no qualms about choosing their own lovers. In this respect Cleopatra was a typical Egyptian woman of her time. Egyptian men described sex as "knowing a woman perfectly" and typically treated their women with kind consideration, appropriate to a partner with whom one would share what they considered to be life's supreme "joy."

Cleopatra had a gift for unforgettable entrances, winning Julius Caesar's favor when she arrived at his feet, unrolled in a rug. After Caesar was murdered, she had both her country's interests and her children with Caesar to protect from the rapacious appetite of the expanding Roman Empire. Knowing that Marc Antony had recently declared himself the new Dionysus, incarnate god of revelry and wine, she had the royal barge washed down with rose water and the sails soaked in the heady fragrance of camphire and then sailed out to meet Rome's best-known warrior in the port town of Tarsus. Dressed in a diaphanous gown of "cloth-of-gold," her skin was gleaming like polished marble, dusted with a special powder made of ground mother-of-pearl. She surrounded herself with smiling boy "cupids," who fanned her where she lay in her pavilion, a living tableau of Aphrodite, risen from the waves. Cleopatra, who was generally assumed to be divine and immortal anyway, was, as far as the observing crowd was concerned, the love goddess incarnate. Like Isis, the ancient Egyptian goddess, she came wrapped in an enchanting, all-encompassing aroma. She could not be resisted; everyone in the civilized world knew that it was pointless to attempt to escape a goddess's will. There was only one thing that could happen when the goddess of love and the god of wine came together: according to common belief, the two were the parents of Priapus, the Roman phallic god of lust. Once Cleopatra set such forces in motion, Antony had no choice but to submit.

Living in Alexandria, then hub of the civilized world, Cleopatra had access to the finest fragrance materials available in the world. Alexandria was an intensely fragrant place in which statues of gods and goddesses were wreathed with scented flowers and anointed every morning with perfumes to fortify them for a day of worship and supplications, in a ritual known as the "opening of mouths and eyes." When the sun set, *kyphi*, a soothing, aromatic compound of cinnamon, spikenard, peppermint, juniper, and myrrh, among many other ingredients, was burned. It was later adopted by the Greeks and Romans as an aromatic and medicinal and was described by Plutarch as having the ability to "lull to sleep, allay anxieties, and brighten the dreams." Alexandria remained the world's center of aromatic trade for another sixteen hundred years after Cleopatra's death. Even today, Egypt is one of the great essential oil-producing countries.

In Cleopatra's time, cinnamon, costus root, spikenard, lemongrass, ginger, pepper, and sandalwood were imported from the East along trade routes established fifteen hundred years earlier by the Egyptian queen Hatshepsut, who traded copper and turquoise for sandalwood and aromatic "incense" trees for her royal gardens. Egyptians loved gardens, favoring above all the narcotic-scented blue water lily, or blue lotus. The heads of this flower, which contained a hallucinogenic substance, were steeped in wine to create a mind-altering beverage. Also popular were the white Madonna lily, which the Egyptians distilled, the cistus, and the henna flower, or camphire, which Cleopatra used to scent her sails.

Perfumes and ointments were concocted in special laboratories by priests in the temples. Egyptian women washed often with scented toilet waters and wore cones of perfumed fat on their heads to keep their skin oiled and fragrant in the intense, dry heat of the desert. They wore jewelry made of fragrant gums and scented woods that released sweet aromas when heated by the warmth of the skin.

The woman who knew how to make an entrance knew how to make an exit as well. Not quite forty, Cleopatra found herself a prisoner of the new Roman emperor Octavian, following Antony's defeat and death. She knew what was in store for her if she were to be taken back to Rome as a captive. She would be paraded through the streets, naked and in chains, and thoroughly humiliated before being publicly beaten and killed. Appearing resigned to her fate, she paid a last visit to Antony's grave, wreathing it with fragrant flowers and kissing it passionately. Afterward, she and her most trusted women, Iras and Charmian, were allowed to go, under guard, to the main chamber of the mausoleum. Cleopatra ordered a bath and had her hair dressed and scented with jasmine. Attired as the goddess Isis, she ate a sumptuous meal. Then, after allowing herself to be bitten by an asp hidden in a basket of dessert figs, she laid down upon a bed of pure gold and, wrapped in a cloud of fragrance, died.

Beauty and the Bath

OKAY, SO NOT EVERY WOMAN feels ready to metamorphose into a seductive siren at a moment's notice. The spirit may be willing, but chances are the flesh is frazzled from a long day at work, or running around after one or more overactive kids, or maybe both. An aromatic bath provides the perfect transition place to reawaken the senses and to soothe exhaustion and fatigue.

A twenty-minute soak in a tub with nine drops of **lavender** added to warm (not hot!) water can melt even the most stubborn nervous tension. A few drops of precious **rose, jasmine**, or **neroli** in the bathwater take away all but pleasant thoughts of love. Two drops each of **frankincense, benzoin**, and **sandalwood** warm up a body that is cold from fatigue and tension and remind you to breathe! But when you've really had it and you just can't miss that important date or dinner, banish fatigue and mental cobwebs with this rejunevating blend:

THE "I CAN'T TAKE IT ANYMORE" BATH

3 drops **juniper**
5 drops **rosemary**
2 drops **frankincense**

Swish the oils around thoroughly before you get in. May cause redness or warming to sensitive skin, but the mental clarity and improved mood are worth the slight discomfort!

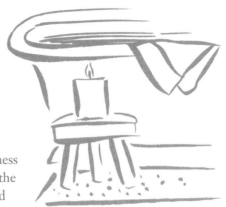

@

Part of being an esscentual woman is to create your own definitions of words like "beautiful" and "sexy." Movie stars and supermodels in our culture occupy a place very similar to the Greco-Roman gods and goddesses. They personify certain attributes and qualities and are every bit as petulant, temperamental, and entertaining as were the dwellers on Mount Olympus to their devotees. But they're not "real"! It takes an army of attendants and high priests of hair, makeup, wardrobe, and lighting to make women look like they do on billboards, in movies, or on the pages of fashion magazines. The rest of us mere mortals must make do with what we can do for ourselves, and that's where essential oils are truly invaluable.

Beauty, of course, doesn't really come in a bottle, as so many cosmetic ads seem to promise. The contents of the bottle are, at best, only a means to an end. Cosmetics are meant to enhance what's already there, not to create something that doesn't exist. True feminine beauty starts from the inside, with proper nutrition and good health and enough exercise to keep your system toned and running smoothly.

Beauty is your innate sense of who you really are, the cultivation and appreciation of what is special and unique about you, and you alone. A woman who knows who she is, who keeps both feet firmly planted in her own womanliness, regardless of cultural stereotypes, is beautiful, sexy, and practically irresistible!

That said, let's get back to externals. Once you've beautified your inner attitude, take a moment to evaluate the largest organ you present to the world: your skin.

Most of what we've learned about the protective fabric of cells that separates what's outside of ourselves from what is within has been discovered in the last fifty years. The good news is that whatever condition your skin is in, it can be improved, for skin has a marvelous ability to regenerate itself. About a million dead skin cells are shed every hour that you're alive, and two new layers of skin are forming every four hours or so. Through exfoliation of old skin and nourishing the newly developing cells, the texture and sensitivity of your "outer cloak" can be greatly enhanced. Taking good care of your skin makes you look more radiant and feel more alive, increasing your sexual responsiveness and your lover's enjoyment of you as well.

Use rose hip seed oil (also known as *rosa mosqueta*) in your body and massage blends to repair and rejuvenate your skin at its deepest levels. All the natural nut oils have nourishing and emollient effects on the skin, though hazelnut, macadamia, sweet almond, shea, and pecan are my personal favorites. **Lavender**, **blue chamomile**, and **helichrysm** are soothing and regenerating to skin cells; **rose**, **jasmine**, **sandalwood**, and **frankincense** replenish moisture and improve elasticity. Oily skin can benefit from the sebum-balancing properties of **geranium**, **palmarosa**, and **ylang-ylang**.

To reduce the appearance of cellulite and to keep your skin always in tiptop condition, use a natural-bristle body brush before every bath or shower, starting at the soles of the feet, brushing upward toward the heart, and staying away from the too-sensitive areas of breasts, neck, and face. A drop of **cypress**, **juniper**, **rosemary**, **lemon**, **eucalyptus**, or **lemongrass** added to the bristles gives a boost to circulation and can help expedite the elimination of excess fluids. The same essences can also be used in the bath and in body oils.

After dry brushing, rehydrate tired skin to a satiny, glowing finish that begs to be touched with a scented bath oil.

"TOUCH ME" BATH OIL

¼ cup oil
1 cup rose, orange blossom, or chamomile floral water
2 tbsp. liquid glycerin
30–40 drops essential oil of your choice

Mix all ingredients in a glass bottle or jar and shake well to mix. Add a drop of food coloring if desired. Shake thoroughly before using, as the ingredients will separate when left standing. One recipe is enough for about four baths.

Massaging Him

We touch heaven when we lay our hands on a human body.

NOVALIS, 1772

WOMEN OFTEN COMPLAIN THAT MEN don't express their feelings, but in actuality, men are expressing them all the time. They just do it in a different language. Because females develop verbal and language skills earlier and more rapidly, women start to talk to each other about how they feel when they are very young. Boys and men tend to express their emotions more in body language and physical actions.

Complicating matters even further is the fact that part of the acculturation process for men involves the control and suppression of powerful drives and feelings. Men have a greater proportion of muscle mass than women and therefore an even greater tendency to "body armoring," in which suppressed feelings are held as tension and rigidity in the muscles and connective tissues of the body. While body armoring successfully prevents negative or overwhelming feelings from entering consciousness, it locks out enjoyable sensations at the same time, narrowing the range of possible emotional experience. Inflexibility and numbness are the inevitable result. A bodyworker I know has commented on this phenomenon by describing one well-armored male client as "a big knot covered with skin."

So here's my advice: If you love him, rub him! Regular massage will slowly dissolve armoring and release any backlog of emotional tension being held in the body. Often a man will become more centered, peaceful, and emotionally expressive as the old armor is stripped away. Comforting essential oils such as **benzoin**, **rose**, **geranium**, **mandarin**, **melissa**, and **marjoram** can greatly enhance the process. (The Rose Petal Caress massage oil included in your kit is a perfect blend for this purpose.) Plenty of nurturing, nonsexual touch and the sharing of feelings are as important to a love relationship as sexual contact. The wider the range of feelings you are able to express and experience with each other, the more intimate and powerful your lovemaking will be.

Instructions for a great back rub are included in the next chapter. Because men tend to focus their tensions in the lower back and buttocks, add the following strokes.

LOWER BACK SPIRALS. Warm a teaspoon or so of aromatic oil in your hands, then smooth it over the buttocks and lower back. Starting at the top of the crack between the buttocks, use your thumbs to make small spirals upward along either side of the tailbone to the top of the sacrum, then press your thumbs along the top of the hips and move them out, across and down the side of the body to the floor. Repeat several times.

THUMBS OVER THE MOUNTAIN. Use a few big, kneading strokes to loosen up the muscles before you begin, using more oil if necessary, but not too much, because you'll be working next with your thumbs. Starting at the bottom, press your thumbs firmly into the flesh of the buttocks and follow the curve up, around, and down the side of the hips. Use as much pressure as your lover can comfortably tolerate; this can be a tender and sensitive area. Return to the first position and move your thumbs apart slightly to describe a second curved line that is parallel to and outside the first, continuing until you have no curve left to follow. Repeat several times. (Men: This is a great stroke for women, too!)

REDISTRIBUTING THE ENERGY. Now that you've freed up some of the emotional energy that was trapped in body tension, you'll want to redirect it into the rest of the body, where it can be reabsorbed or released. Place your hand on your lover's lower back to one side of the spine, palm down, fingers flat and pointing toward the shoulders. Using firm and even pressure, press down and move the hand slowly up toward the top of the spine, with the other hand following right behind. Visualize that with the pressure you are moving his energy up and out of the lower back into the rest of his body. Repeat several times, then do the same thing on the other side of the spine.

Emotional Ups and Downs: Taking Care of Yourself

INTENSELY EMOTIONAL UPS AND DOWNS often accompany deepening intimacy. There's something deeply comforting about being enveloped in warm, womblike, scented bath water that can help to soothe the turbulence inside.

While every woman is different, if we study ourselves we're likely to find certain patterns to our emotional outbursts, well-worn paths of feeling we tend to travel when we're off-balance or spiraling downward into a negative state. Some of us tend toward anxiety, others to anger, still others to depression as a front-line response. Essential oils can nip a negative emotional state in the bud, derailing the well-worn response and giving you the freedom to choose whether or not that's how you want to continue to feel at any given moment.

Of course, a bathtub isn't always handy when you get upset! If you know the ways in which you're most likely to feel and express emotional distress, it may help to carry one or two small vials of essential oil with you in your purse, to be taken out and sniffed as necessary. You can put a drop of chosen essence on the back of your hand or just under your nose (choose nonirritating oils if you'll be using them undiluted), which has the added bonus of reminding you to breathe. There are also vials or flasks that can be filled with your favorite essences and worn around your neck as jewelry, where they're always within easy reach. Fill them with a single oil, or create your own blend.

Calming, cooling **lavender** can be used for many "first aid" situations, both emotional and physical. **Ylang-ylang** helps to dissipate anger. **Clary sage** is a euphoric, for those who tend to weepy depression. All the **citruses** are sunny and help to dispel the dark clouds of anxiety and fear, and **mandarin** has a mild tranquilizing effect as well. **Jasmine** and **bay laurel** improve confidence. Feeling touchy, a little spaced-out and hypersensitive? Try a grounding oil such as **vetiver**, perhaps with an added drop of **patchouli** and **orange**. **Angelica** and **juniper** dispel negativity. **Frankincense** helps to leave the past behind, such as when you're starting a new relationship and can't stop thinking about the last one you left. For obsessive thinking or excessive preoccupation with a new love, to the degree that you're having difficulty focusing on the rest of your life, get out of your head with a grounding or centering essence, such as **vetiver**, **spikenard**, **myrrh**, or **sandalwood**. If you're having trouble speaking up for yourself or telling your lover what you need, use **chamomile** or **rose**.

Sometimes too much of a good thing is just that: too much. Hitting a wall or ceiling in your capacity for intimacy often manifests as a pointless argument, a feeling of impending illness, or as sudden, inexplicable disinterest in your lover, a "frozen heart." What may really be going on is that you just need a little space, to reset your boundaries and regain a feeling of emotional equilibrium. Allow yourself some quiet time, away from everybody and everything, and try this blend, added to a bath. (Or add the essential oils to two ounces of massage oil, and bring the blend with you to be used during a one-hour, full body massage. Try it! It can work wonders.)

THE "I NEED SOME SPACE" BLEND

6 drops marjoram
18 drops lavender
1 drop peppermint

Mix, and allow the oils to integrate for at least half an hour before using. Enough for two baths, or for two ounces of massage oil.

Sensual Perfumes

With their soft hips covered with beautiful fabrics and trappings,
their breasts perfumed with sandalwood, covered with necklaces and jewels,
and with hair perfumed from the bath, the beautiful women coax
their lovers to burning desire.

RITUSANHARA, *classic love poem of India*

A WOMAN EXPECTS A LOT FROM A PERFUME. First, it must have a pleasing and provocative fragrance, not only in the bottle but also on her skin. It should make her feel good: beautiful, sexy, and alluring. The scent then goes forth from her as a kind of sexual lure, irresistibly drawing a chosen man's attention, causing him to desire to be closer to her. This drawing closer should ultimately result in an embrace or physical contact, during which subtle vestiges of her scent are left on the lover, on skin, clothes, or bedsheets, to conjure later fond memories. Certain essences or absolutes can be generally relied on for their aphrodisiac properties, such as **jasmine**, **rose**, **tuberose**, **narcissus**, **neroli**, and **sandalwood**.

Once you've embarked on a relationship, you have the added advantage of being able to create a perfume that appeals specifically to your lover. Try offering various essences for your lover to smell and rate on a sexiness scale of one to ten. When blending the new perfume, use your lover's top-ranked essences as dominant notes.

Of Mistresses and Queens

AROMATHERAPY FOR LOVERS, like perfume, is about enhancing love, creating emotionally charged memories, and conditioning the arousal response. Mistresses throughout history have understood this all too well. A mistress's position in her lover's affections depended on her beauty, charm, and ability to seduce and please; it was not, like the role of a wife or a queen, guaranteed, protected, or upheld by law.

Some queens, like Elizabeth I of England, dealt with the difficult issues of kings and their mistresses by simply avoiding the issue of marriage altogether. The favorite perfume of the Virgin Queen, a blend of **benzoin** and antiaphrodisiac **marjoram**, likely helped her to keep her resolve. Some claimed the sudden interest she developed in fragrance and perfume in the fourteenth year of her reign had something to do with her fondness for Edward de Vere, Duke of Oxford, who presented her with a pair of scented gloves. History is mum on the subject of whether or not they were really lovers, but it is interesting to note that there was no perfume industry in England at all until after the Duke's treasured gift.

While it's tempting to think that the "wife/mistress," "whore/madonna" view of women's sexuality originated with Christian beliefs that separated flesh and spirit, it actually began much earlier, in ancient Greece. There, good wives were "fields to be plowed" and, with daughters, were kept cloistered at home, rarely seen on the streets or at public functions. Instead, when men wanted to go out to the theater or to a party, they went accompanied by hetairai, Greek courtesans who lived by their wits and beauty, with a heavy dose of the right perfumes. A typical courtesan, preparing for an evening out with her lover, would begin with a full body massage given by slaves, followed by a scented bath. After being dried by swan feathers (swans were sacred to the love goddess Aphrodite) she would then be rubbed all over with scented oils. **Myrrh** was a favorite fragrance among hetairai.

The royal mistress was a fixture, something of a status symbol, and certainly an arbiter of fashion among the European courts. Diana of Poitiers, mistress of Francis I during the 16th century, was also the leading patroness of perfume of her time. Known for her legendary youth and beauty, she was the king's lover for more than thirty years. Her beauty and allure still very much intact after Francis's death, she then became mistress of his successor, Henry II.

Jeanne Antoinette Poisson, the marquise de Pompadour, was so beautiful as a child that an old woman was inspired to prophesy she would one day be mistress to a king. Her impressionable family set about preparing the little girl for her future, and she did indeed catch the eye of the French monarch Louis XV. She was known for her exquisite taste, and the art of French perfumery evolved from a craft to an industry during her patronage. Madame de Pompadour kept her favorite scents in six rock crystal bottles, with a matching coffee cup and *bonbonnière* to revive her flagging energies after the rigors of her toilette. At Choisy, only one of the many chateaus she occupied with the king, she spent 500,000 livres a year on perfumes. The "beauty spot" was one of the fashion fads she started, originating in a game she played with the king, during which he had to search her lovely body to find where she had concealed tiny patches. At first worried that her temperament was too "cold" to satisfy her lover on a continuing basis, she ate libido-enhancing dishes such as chocolate prepared with ambergris and vanilla, truffles, and celery soup.

Later, she solved the dilemma by establishing a garden of young virgins from which the king could freely choose, and kept herself busy with running his kingdom. Madame de Pompadour's favorite scents were **rose**, **lavender**, **millefleur**, and **hyacinth**. She also used **orange blossom water** as a perfume and cosmetic.

Five years after the marquise de Pompadour died, the king took a second mistress. The comtesse Du Barry was a common woman of the streets, who was said to have a complexion like "rose leaves dipped in cream." She loved the clean, fresh smell of the original *eau de cologne* made from a combination of grape spirits, **neroli**, **bergamot**, **lavender**, and **rosemary**, and spent a fortune on it. Comtesse Du Barry died by the guillotine during the French Revolution, as did Marie Antoinette, who loved the light fragrances of violet and rose water.

Another victim of the guillotine was the first husband of the empress Josephine, who married Napoleon in a civil ceremony in 1796. Josephine, the Creole daughter of an Orleans merchant, grew up on the island of Martinique, where women preserved their beauty by massaging coconut and almond creams into the skin daily. Josephine was especially fond of the scents of **violet**, **musk**, **hyacinth**, and **mignonette**. Napoleon also gave her Spanish **jasmine** as a gift. After her husband marched on Cairo, Josephine popularized the bare-armed, semi-Egyptian look with the white Empire gown, accented with patchouli-scented paisley shawls handmade in India. To keep your skin as fragrant, smooth, and luminous as that of Napoleon's empress, try the following:

CREME JOSEPHINE

1–2 oz. coconut oil
10 drops jasmine absolute
10 drops sandalwood

Warm the coconut oil, which tends to solidify at room temperature, just until it liquefies. Mix in the jasmine and sandalwood. Pour into a small, flat cosmetic or sachet jar and allow to set. Use as a skin softener or creme perfume. The coconut oil liquefies quickly under the heat of your fingertips. Keep in the refrigerator during very hot weather.

Even stodgy Queen Victoria had a favorite perfume, Essence des Bouquets, which included a few aphrodisiac essences. Queen Alexandra loved **white rose**, which is still grown and distilled in Bulgaria today. Alexandra's sister, the Czarina of Russia, was fond of *chypre*, a soft, sexy blend of **oakmoss, sandalwood**, and **bergamot**, which is named for the island of Cyprus, where Aphrodite was said to have washed ashore.

The very first alcoholic perfume was created in 1370, based on the essence of **rosemary**, according to a recipe given to Queen Elizabeth of Hungary by a mysterious hermit who told her that by using it, she would keep her beauty intact until her death. It is assumed that the perfume performed as promised, because she was still fielding proposals of marriage at the age of seventy-two. Hungary Water is meant to be used as a body splash and can also be added to the bath. (**Caution: Do not drink this or any other mixture containing essential oils described in this book!** Essential oils taken internally can have a damaging effect on the liver and internal organs, and should never be ingested without the guidance of a qualified physician.)

HUNGARY WATER

1 qt. alcohol (grape spirits or ethyl alcohol if you can get them, high-proof brandy or vodka if you can't)

150 drops rosemary

75 drops melissa

75 drops lemon

2 drops peppermint

A few drops each rose and neroli (optional)

8 oz. rose water

8 oz. orange blossom water

Add the essential oils to the alcohol in a half-gallon-size glass bottle or jar, swirl to blend, and allow to sit overnight, or for a few days if you're patient enough! Then add the rose water and orange blossom water, and shake well. Keep in the refrigerator for an excellent cooling splash for summer. Apply with cotton balls as a facial toner or cleanser. Splash some in the bath for an invigorating pick-me-up. Always shake well before using.

True **melissa**, or **lemon balm**, is extremely expensive and rare. If you can't find it (or afford it!), try extracting the essence in the alcohol first, using the fresh herb, which grows fairly easily in a garden or pot. Make sure the herb is clean and dry. Fill a jar with lemon balm leaves, top with alcohol and put into a dark cupboard for two weeks, shaking daily. Then remove the herbs and strain the alcohol through a coffee filter. It should have a sweet, light, lemony aroma.

When all is said and done, what does it mean to be an "esscentual woman"? Be fragrant! Live like a flower, like a queen, like a goddess of love, emanating a divine aroma in everything that you do! The essences you use create an aura of beauty and elegance around everything you touch. Scent your home, your clothing, yourself! The use of essential oils can transform daily tasks from meaningless drudgery to small but important and beautiful acts of grace and love. Aromatherapy for lovers is not something to be kept in the bedroom and brought out only for special occasions. Every day, every moment is an "esscentual" opportunity.

FIVE

The Esscentual Man

Woman is like a fruit, which will not yield its sweetness until you
rub it between your hands. Look at the basil plant; if you don't
rub it warm with your fingers it will not emit any scent . . .
It is the same with woman.

FROM *The Perfumed Garden*

IF YOU REALLY WANT TO MAKE AN IMPRESSION on a woman, if you want to be the best lover she ever had, it's very simple: Touch her! And talk to her, too! Women require a little conversation and a lot of touching to get fully turned on. Men, whose erotic arousal process starts visually, often fail to understand why they don't get an immediate response when they give the object of their desire a come-hither look and then pounce. Well, now you know. It's a biological difference. It's that oxytocin thing that's covered in chapter 1. Touching and kissing a woman are crucial to building in her a high level of sexual arousal and enjoyment (more on why this is so in the next chapter).

Some men know this instinctively. Two thousand years ago, Marc Antony was harassed by some of his more macho contemporaries for giving foot rubs, considered the duty of a slave, to Cleopatra, but the Roman warrior knew what he was doing. Egypt's glamorous and wealthy queen remained devoted to him for more than ten years, long after his youthful glory had faded, until they were parted by death. **Ylang-ylang**, with a few drops of **orange** added, is a perfect foot rub combination, possessing a sweet and somewhat sneaky seductive punch.

When you've progressed beyond the foot rub stage, make a point of including sensual massage in your seduction ritual. Use an oil containing your lover's favorite "turn-on" essences (**jasmine**, **rose**, and **neroli** are expensive but pretty reliable in this regard), or use one of the Aromatherapy for Lovers massage blends included in your kit for optimal results.

The Esscentual Back Rub

WOMEN TEND TO CONCENTRATE BODILY TENSION in the neck, shoulders, and upper back. The resulting tight, heavy feelings contribute to a sense that the weight of the world is on their shoulders, which is not a very sexy way to feel! The trapezius muscles, which run from the neck outward to the shoulders, can be so tense at times that having them touched or kneaded will be painful at first. Start with gentle pressure, and increase it if your lover is comfortable with your doing so. Use only a small amount of oil, a teaspoon or so. You want to lubricate the skin just enough for the movements; too much and your partner will be too slippery to handle. (We'll do that on purpose in the next chapter, however.) Rub the massage oil in the palms of your hands to warm it up before it touches her skin. (Cold oil poured on the back will quickly produce about twice as much tension as was there before you started!)

1. THE WELCOMING PRESS. Begin with your lover lying face down. Straddling her or kneeling at her side, press gently down on her shoulders, on either side of her spine. NEVER PRESS DIRECTLY ON THE SPINE DURING A MAS-SAGE, as you can easily dislocate spinal vertebrae in this way. Give her a few moments to get used to the feeling of your hands on her skin. Then start the back-warmer stroke.

2. THE BACKWARMER: UP, ACROSS, AND DOWN. In the backwarmer, you'll be doing just that: warming the back. The friction from the stroking brings blood to the surface of the skin, which increases circulation and helps the essential oils begin to penetrate the skin on either side of the torso and along the spinal column, where so many of the body's nerve endings and blood vessels are located. The movement is up, around, and down: with a flat hand, fingers together, palm in contact with her skin, move the hands in parallel lines up either side of the spine, then out and across the shoulders, and down the sides of the torso. If the pressure is too light, she may feel ticklish on the sides of her body. You want a firm, reassuring touch here, to let her know she's in good hands.

3. KNEADING. Working as deeply as is comfortable for your lover, use your fingers to knead the muscles of the back, starting with the neck and shoulders and working your way down. As her muscles loosen and relax, her back will become softer and more pliable. That's a sign that you're doing a great job. Encourage her to let you know what feels good and where she wants extra attention. Use more oil as necessary.

4. RAKING. Spread your fingers and, keeping them somewhat stiff, rake them down the back from shoulders to buttocks. This feels wonderful when it's properly done and releases deeper, underlying tissue tensions.

5. LOWER BACK, BUTTOCKS, AND THIGHS. The lower back and sacrum (the downward-pointing triangle located between the buttocks at the end of the spine) can become congested and tender, especially in premenstrual women. Lightly massage this area with small, circular strokes, then continue with kneading strokes on buttocks, hips, and upper thighs.

Once you get to your lover's thighs, you may find yourself getting distracted and decide to shift your focus to other kinds of touching! Or you may want to try out some massage strokes of your own design on any areas that don't feel fully relaxed. Or you can ask your partner to turn over and continue the massage with a few more strokes to the front of the body.

6. SHOULDER AND CHEST PRESSES. Kneeling behind your partner, as she is lying face up, press down on her shoulders and hold. Tell her to take a deep, releasing breath, and let the essential oils in the massage blend work their magic as you increase the pressure of your hands slightly. At the end of her exhalation, release. Slide your hands up and over her clavicle, or collar bone, and press gently. Have her take a deep breath as you hold, then release. Move your hands to the center of her chest, between her breasts, and laying one hand atop the other like a sandwich, press gently, have her take a deep breath, and release.

7. SEXUAL ENERGY RELEASE POINTS, NECK AND EARS. Encourage her to breathe in a deep and relaxing manner as you gently massage her neck, making small circles over the release points on the upper neck and about halfway up the ears. If the massage is a prelude to lovemaking, now is a really good time to let the kissing begin. Remember too that a woman's breasts are highly charged with erotic energy and can create a dramatic arousal response when massaged or caressed.

8. IMPROVISE! You're on your own from here. I have a feeling that you'll do just fine.

Bathing Together

*For flavor, instant sex will never supersede
the stuff you have to peel and cook.*

QUENTIN CRISP

BATHING TOGETHER, if you have a nice, big bathtub, can be very romantic. Light a candle for atmosphere (most bathroom light is too harsh to be seductive) and place it well away from the tub, as the flame will otherwise quickly burn off the aromatic vapors of essential oil you add to the water. A drop or two of **jasmine** (with **cedar** or **sandalwood**, if desired) or **ylang-ylang** (possibly with a few added drops of **tangerine**, **mandarin**, or **orange**) creates a sexy scentual aura around you both. Stimulating **patchouli** has an earthy, exotic smell and blends well with **orange** or **rose**, the latter of which gives a loving note to sensuality. **Rose** by itself aids relaxation and expansive thoughts of love. Add **benzoin** or **vanilla** for warmth. A few drops of **clary sage** can bring out smiles and giggles. (Don't overdo the latter, and don't use in conjunction with alcohol. You might get bigger laughs out of a bigger dose, but a big headache is likely to follow!)

For really deep relaxation try **neroli**, which blends well with **petitgrain**, **tangerine** or **mandarin**, and **sandalwood**. **Lavender** is soothing and balancing, though not particularly sexy. Try spicing it up with some **bergamot**, **geranium**, and euphoric **clary sage**. To get out of your head and into your body, use grounding **vetiver** or **myrrh**. Conversely, if you're feeling heavy and want to lighten up, try a few drops of **balsam fir**, or a blend of **jasmine** with **orange** and **frankincense**.

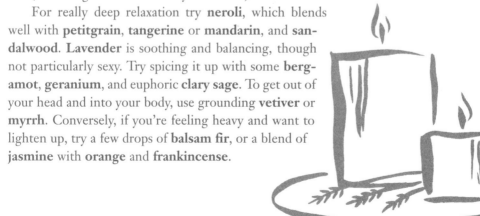

A single drop of **peppermint** with **tangerine** makes a tingly and refreshing before-love bath for a hot summer night. A little bit of spice, such as **ginger, cinnamon**, or **nutmeg**, warms a cold winter evening and revs up the libido. (**Caution: Spice oils can be irritating to the skin.** Dilute one or two drops in a milder essence, such as rosewood or lavender, or in a teaspoon of milk or oil before adding to the bath water. **Discontinue use if skin irritation results.**)

When you've found the woman of your dreams, treat her like a love goddess with the following bath blend of Nature's most precious essences. The formula is inspired by and named for the secret bathing perfume used by the goddesses on Mount Olympus, which made them irresistible to mortals and immortals alike!

AMBROSIA

3 drops jasmine
3 drops rose
3 drops neroli
3 drops sandalwood

Fill the tub with comfortably warm water. Add the essences, swishing gently with your hand to mix. Invite her in.

The Scented Male in History

He must get up early in the morning, answer the calls of nature,
wash his teeth, smear his body with just a little fragrant paste,
inhale fragrant smoke, wear some flower, just give the lips a rub
with wax and red juice, look at his face in the mirror, chew betel
leaves along with some mouth deodorants, and then attend to his work.

from the KAMA SUTRA, *ca. a.d. 400, describing the life of the*
typical high caste Hindu man

DESPITE THE IMPRESSION most guys give of agreeing with the ancient Roman wit Martial, who sardonically observed "He that smells always well seldom does so," prominent men throughout history have often additionally distinguished themselves through their lavish use of perfume. Ever since Pluto lured Persephone into the underworld with the intoxicating fragrance of the narcissus flower, created just for that purpose by his big brother Zeus, men have employed scents for their seductive effects on women, as well as for healthful benefits and personal or aesthetic enjoyment.

The Hanging Gardens of Babylon, considered one of the Seven Wonders of the ancient world, were actually an aromatic labor of love. The Babylonian king Nebuchadnezzar created them to cheer up his homesick wife, Amytes, who missed the fragrant lilies and other plants of her homeland in Medea. Medean men were notorious for their use of perfumes, a fondness they passed on to their Assyrian conquerors, who spent hours each day braiding their beards with fragrant oils.

The power of a pleasing fragrance to transform an otherwise ordinary man into an irresistible love object is not just a fabrication of Madison Avenue advertising executives trying to sell aftershave. The idea actually goes back thousands of years, to an ancient Greco-Roman myth, in which an exceptionally ugly boat pilot named

Phaon unknowingly transports the love goddess Venus to her birthplace on the island of Cyprus. Venus is so delighted with Phaon's navigational skill that she gives him a mysterious perfume elixir, which transforms him into a beautiful youth. Sappho later falls in love with Phaon, who doesn't return her affections, which inspires the poetess to throw herself off an oceanside promontory at Leucadia, a Greek lover's leap said to cure the heart of unrequited passions. It cured Sappho's permanently.

The Greek ruler Antiochus "the Mad," scourge of the ancient Hebrews, was perhaps history's greatest aromatic party animal. After sacking Jerusalem and installing a statue of Zeus in the temple, he held a huge sports meet, livened up by two hundred topless cheerleaders who ran through the crowd with golden sprinklers, dousing spectators and athletes with precious perfumes. As irony would have it, King Solomon, builder of the temple that Antiochus desecrated, was himself perhaps the most esscentual man who ever lived, if the erotic, perfume-soaked imagery of his Song of Songs is any indication.

Alexander the Great, who sat and wept when he realized there were no worlds left for him to conquer, comforted himself with the aromas of perfumes sprinkled throughout his apartments, and the fragrant smoke of burning resins such as **frankincense** and **myrrh**. Alexander also collected specimens of fragrant plants during his world exploits, which he sent home to his school chum Theophrastus, author of the first known treatise on scent, "Concerning Odors."

The men of ancient Athens gathered at perfume shops in much the same way that men converge in coffee shops or cafes today. Greek men were famous for using a different perfume on each part of the body and favored a scent called Susinum, which was a blend of **rose**, **cinnamon**, and **myrrh**. Scents were used to greet visitors and to entertain, as at the ancient Greek dinner party described in this excerpt from the "Settler of Alexis":

He slipp'd four doves, whose wings were saturate
With scents, all different in kind—each bird
Bearing its own appropriate sweets—these doves
Wheeling in circles round, let fall upon us
A shower of sweet perfumery.

The Roman emperor Caligula's use of perfume was as excessive as his sexual appetites, and he depended heavily on aromatic baths and massages to revitalize him after his debauches. Nero likewise disguised his body odor with fragrant oils. Rooms devoted to aromatic massage were an important feature in the massive public baths he constructed in Rome, moving Martial to remark "What is worse than Nero? What is better than Nero's baths?" The ceiling of one of the dining rooms in his palatial Golden House was fitted with silver spouts that sprayed scented waters and perfumes over his guests. At his wife Poppaea's funeral, Nero burned more incense than Arabia could produce in ten years.

After the fall of the Roman Empire, scents became too rare and costly for the average citizen and were reserved primarily for use by rulers and in the newly established Catholic church. Charlemagne had a great fondness for perfumes, which were an important feature of his elegant court. Knights of the Crusades bathed in rose petals, having brought back the habit of fragrant living from their sojourns in the East. The use of scent reached a heyday in Europe under the Sun King, Louis XIV. His court at Versailles was popularly known as *la cour parfumée*, because a different perfume was used there every single day.

The self-declared emperor Napoleon went through up to six hundred bottles of "Water of Cologne" each year, using the blend of **rosemary**, **neroli**, and **bergamot** essences externally for fragrance and personal hygiene, and internally as well. (The eau de cologne used by Napoleon is still made today by Roget et Gallet, according to the recipe originated by Giovanni Maria Farina's uncle Feminis' original formula.) Because the alcohol used for perfumes was not denatured in those days, favorite scents often doubled as medicinal liquors, due to the healing properties of their fragrant essential oils, an early form of aromatherapy.

Indeed, the term "aromatherapy" was coined by a man, René Maurice Gattefossé, a French cosmetic chemist. Other prominent male pioneers in the development of modern aromatherapy include Dr. Jean Valnet, Dr. Daniel Penoel, Dr. Daniel Lapraz, Pierre Franchomme, and Dietrich Gumbel. Here in the United States, knowledge and accessibility of aromatherapy and essential oils have been greatly increased by men such as Marcel Lavabre of Aroma Vera, aromatic researcher John Steele, and aromatherapy educators Michael Scholes and Dr. Kurt Schnaubelt.

Daily Esscentuals

IT'S EASY TO BECOME A MORE ESSCENTUAL MAN by incorporating essential oils into your daily regime. Vials of your favorite essences can be kept handy in the medicine cabinet for daily use. A few drops of **lavender**, applied neat (undiluted) to just-shaved skin makes a simple and effective aftershave treatment. Its cell-rejuvenating properties help heal minor cuts and abrasions quickly, and the aroma is attractive and fresh, appropriate to a day at the office or an evening out.

Essences can be added to unscented shower gels to give an aromatic start to any day.

Rosemary, **basil**, **eucalyptus**, **lemon,** and **peppermint**, singly or in any combination, clear the mind and wake up the body. Try adding a drop or two of any of the above essences to your shampoo or conditioner before applying it to your hair, and you'll carry the aroma with you all day long.

At the gym, essential oils can be taken into the steam room or sauna and rubbed into moist skin for their stimulating or revivifying effects after a workout.

If your skin is sensitive, dilute the essence first in an oil carrier (see chapter 2 for dilutions and blending tips). **Bay laurel** gives a heady feeling of confidence and power. **Lime** is stimulating and refreshing, as is **bergamot. (Caution: Never use bergamot on exposed skin before going out into the sun, as it can cause permanent pigment discoloration.) Sandalwood** and **cedar** have woody, masculine smells; some men I know wear a drop just for the sexy aroma. **Tea tree** protects against fungus such as athlete's foot that may linger and proliferate in public showers.

Because all essential oils are antiseptic and antibacterial to a greater or lesser degree, they also make wonderful deodorants. Many can be tried neat, or to lessen the possibilities of irritation, mix your favorite essences into witch hazel for a deodorant splash and shake thoroughly before using. (Essential oils are not, however, antiperspirants. They only inhibit the growth of the bacteria on the surface of the skin that can cause unpleasant body odor.)

Transform your car into Casanova's carriage by keeping a small, pottery diffusor filled with your favorite aphrodisiac essences secreted somewhere inside. **Jasmine, patchouli,** or **rosemary,** or any of the spice oils, such as **cinnamon, nutmeg, coriander,** or **clove** blended with **citruses,** are good for attracting positive female attention while keeping you alert. You'll want to stay away from sedative aphrodisiac oils like neroli and spikenard while you're driving!

Historically men sprinkled their bedsheets with orris root powder, which served the double purpose of keeping the bed sweet-smelling while imparting a subtle fragrance to their skin. You can get a similar effect by putting a few drops of the essence of your choice on a handkerchief or napkin and placing it between the sheets when you make the bed. The aroma impregnates the bedclothes and will find its way to you as you sleep. Try **ylang-ylang, rose, benzoin,** or **geranium** when you'll have company; or **lavender, mandarin,** and **marjoram** when you know you'll be sleeping alone.

@

What does it really mean to be an esscentual man? Solomon's lover, describing him in the Song of Songs, put it best:

His cheeks are as a bed of spices,
As banks of sweet herbs;
His lips are as lilies, dropping liquid myrrh . . .
His mouth is most sweet;
Yea, he is altogether lovely.

SIX

Esscentual Sex

Wang Ziqiao asked Peng Zu, "What is the essence of human energy?"
Peng Zu replied, "No human energy is more essential than sexual energy. When sex-
ual energy is stifled, the hundred channels become ill; if sexual energy is undeveloped,
it is impossible to propagate. Therefore longevity is all a matter of sexual energy."
FROM *Sex, Health, and Long Life: Manuals of Taoist Practice*
TRANS. BY THOMAS CLEARY

For some, sex leads to sainthood; for others it is the road to hell . . .
all depends on your point of view.
HENRY MILLER, *The World of Sex*

THE ETHERIC AROMAS OF NATURE'S ESSENTIAL OILS have a way of penetrating to
the core of things, gently opening up the mind and emotions to greater possibilities. An important aspect of aromatherapy for lovers is the connecting of this

mental and spiritual process to physical experience, to encourage happier, more satisfying sexual relationships. Erotic energy doesn't have to stay put in the bedroom; it can be channeled outward to enrich and enliven all areas of being. The rosy glow of a happy sex life can extend to brighten and illuminate the whole day. Recent studies have shown that couples who feel sexually satisfied with each other are more likely to stay together. Sexual satisfaction and orgasmic capacity are "esscentual" ingredients to maintaining a joyful marriage or long-term intimate relationship.

The more you and your lover know about each other's sexual nature, the better you'll be able to arouse each other and to communicate your needs and desires. This doesn't mean complaining, or giving orders to your lover about what to do and when. It means having an idea of what your partner will find pleasing, increasing each other's capacity for enjoyment, paying attention to what works and what doesn't, and giving lots of positive reinforcement and feedback. Ignorance is definitely not bliss when it comes to loving relationships. With understanding and communication, both of you are more likely to feel comfortable exploring and expressing your sexuality. If this is done as a game of exploration, it can be very liberating, and a lot of fun!

Tantra

SOME OF THE EXERCISES in this chapter draw on concepts and ideas about erotic energy and its expression that have their origin in the ancient discipline of Tantrism, or Tantra. Like yoga and Buddhism, Tantra was born in India and spread in centuries-long waves of popularity throughout Asia, into China and Japan, until it was repressed during the 13th century. Tantric beliefs and practices influenced the Islamic Sufi love cults, which, with the return of the Crusaders to Europe from the East, gave rise to the troubadors and the veneration of women in the form of

Courtly Love. Tantric overtones are also found in early Gnostic Christianity, which was sometimes called *synesaktism*, or the Way of Shakti.

Tantra's central, most sacred image is "the jewel in the lotus," the *lingam* residing in the *yoni*, the symbolic sexual union of Shiva, the male creative force, with Shakti, the universal feminine energy. Through the expression of love, both mental and physical, the goal of Tantra is ecstasy and enlightenment.

> Once you know the centers of your pleasure, you will be better able to share pleasure with another. This is the whole of the Tantra: that you must perceive what you are through knowing yourself and your pleasures; for only then can you give the pleasure you seek and accept the pleasure given to you.
>
> ASHLEY THIRBY, *TANTRA*

> Not to struggle against one's natural desires, and so to attain longevity, what joy!
>
> THE YELLOW EMPEROR
> 2697–2598 B.C.

The Tantric temple was a highly sensual arena dedicated to awakening the senses and the arousal of desire. The walls were often covered with erotic frescoes, such as those still in existence at the caves of Elephanta near Bombay. Wine and aphrodisiac foods stimulated the libido, and part of the spiritual discipline of foreplay included a wide array of "Tantric perfumes," an early version of aromatherapy for lovers. India being a veritable paradise of fragrant plants and flowers, one of the tantras devotes a whole chapter to *deha ranjana*, a Sanskrit term describing scents used to ensure pleasure in sexual union.

The use of erotic fragrances, aphrodisiac foods, and stimulation of the *marmas*, or erogenous zones, was intended to turn the body into one big organ of exquisite sensitivity, an all-over receptor and transmitter of ecstatic sexual energies. (For a more complete description of the marmas and how to locate and stimulate them, see the next chapter.)

The Esscentual Energy Meld

In the profoundest sense touch is the true language of sex.
ASHLEY MONTAGU, *Touching: The Human Significance of the Skin*

TOUCHING ON ALL LEVELS is the purpose of this deceptively simple body and scent awareness exercise. You'll want to use an old set of sheets or towels on the bed or floor for this one, as the oil may or may not wash out completely.

Begin by getting naked. Anoint each other's heart with a drop of pure essence of **rose** or **geranium** and the third eye area above and between the eyebrows with a drop of **sandalwood**. The heavier partner lies down first, and the lighter partner lies on top. You can both be belly down, if that's most comfortable, or fronts facing, if that feels right. If necessary, position a pillow for the top partner's head to rest on for complete comfort. The partner on the bottom visualizes sinking into the floor or bed as tension flows out of the body. The partner on top sinks into the partner below. It may seem awkward at first, but the more you both relax, the lighter you'll seem and the more comforting the position will start to feel to you both. As the tensions leave your body, feel your subtle energies flowing together as one field, one combined aura that encircles you both. You may want to breathe in rhythm together, matching your breath cycles or taking your "in" breath with your partner's "out" breath. Breathe in the aroma of your loving connection; breathe out anything that stands in the way of your perfect union, letting barriers and negative emotions dissolve, transmuted by the fragrant vapors of the essence you've chosen. Continue this way for at least fifteen to thirty minutes, until you both feel lighter than air.

Now that you have dissolved the boundaries between yourselves, have a little fun as you remind each other of where they are! You can use the Ecstasy Rub or Clouds and Rain massage blend from your *Aromatherapy for Lovers* kit, or a light, euphoric massage blend containing **clary sage** or **grapefruit**. Rub a liberal amount over each other's torso, back, and legs. You need to be well oiled, because you're going to give each other a full body massage—literally! Standing, lying, or rolling together, the object is to give each other a massage using any part of your bodies but your hands. See how many positions you can invent, and how much of your bodies you can keep in contact at any given time. Invent movements together, or allow one partner to lead. You're just not allowed to use your hands for the length of the exercise. (Afterward, you can use them for whatever you like.)

Yoni Anatomy and Essences

The mons veneris of the Mother is the triangle of Aphrodite, the "mound of Venus," the mountain connecting man and woman, earth and sky.

NOR HALL, *The Moon and the Virgin*

MOST MEN could name parts of a car engine more accurately than they could describe the various parts of the female sexual anatomy. While they wouldn't dream of taking a long car trip without checking under the hood to make sure there are plenty of oils and fluids and that everything is in good working order, they might consider approaching a woman in precisely that way. A woman deserves at least as much consideration as a car, and a solid working knowledge of her parts is required to achieve optimal performance!

How many women really understand the responses and processes of their own bodies? If the last experience you had with anatomy was dissecting a frog in biology class, read this section thoroughly.

The pubis is the triangle of hair that covers the mons veneris, or "mount of Venus," a fatty pillow that cushions and protects the pubic bone, dividing into a cleft between the thighs. The labia majora form a kind of curtain, or door, that closes over the vagina. During sexual arousal, these outer lips open and swell as the area engorges with blood. The inner lips, or labia minora, are smooth, pinkish, and hairless, and may change in color during arousal, deepening into shades of purple and red.

The clitoris is actually wishbone shaped and extends down either side of the vaginal cleft. The crown, covered by a protective hood of movable skin, is what most of us think of as the "magic button" that stimulates a woman's sexual response, increasing desire for penetration and ultimately bringing on orgasm. The crown of the clitoris erects when a woman is turned on and can be felt as a hardening knob that can sometimes project from under the soft folds of the hood. It can be stimulated directly by fingertips, lips, tongue, or lingam, or indirectly by movements of penetration into the vagina, or through gentle massage of the "G-spot," a sensitive area located within the vagina about midway between the pubic bone and cervix. The level of sensitivity varies from woman to woman, but continued stimulation of the clitoris, directly or indirectly, will generally result in a climax.

Erotic guidebooks such as the *Kama Sutra* recognize that there are different configurations in women's sexual parts that require different techniques to achieve optimal arousal. The clitoris may be near or far from the vaginal opening; the G-spot may be just inside the vaginal lips, or located deeper inside. Sometimes the shape of the man's lingam fits the yoni perfectly as a key in a lock. More often, lovers need to experiment with a variety of techniques and positions to find what gives maximum pleasure and mutual satisfaction.

Tension, fear, shame, repressed anger, stress, and exhaustion can all interfere with a woman's natural responsiveness, as can genital armoring as a result of inconsiderate lovers, negative or conditioned beliefs, abortions, or unpleasant sexual experiences. Essential oils used in the diffuser, bath, or massage before an amorous interlude help dissolve obstacles to arousal and satisfaction. For women who are having trouble "getting in the mood," be sure to try blends that include the following.

Yoni Essences

Clary sage	Geranium	Jasmine	Lavender
Myrrh	Nutmeg	Palmarosa	Rose
Rosewood	Sandalwood	Spikenard	Ylang-ylang

Lingam Anatomy and Essences

Behold the Shiva Lingam, beautiful as molten gold,
firm as the Himalaya Mountain, tender as a folded leaf,
life-giving like the solar orb; behold the charm
of his sparkling jewels!
from the LINGA PURANA

THE LINGAM IS A FAIRLY SIMPLE ORGAN containing the urethra, the tube through which urine is eliminated from the bladder. The tissues surrounding the urethra engorge with blood during sexual stimulation, resulting in extreme swelling of the glans and penile shaft, popularly known as "erection." Underneath the penile shaft is the scrotum, in which sperm is produced and the testicles are contained. As a man approaches sexual climax, the testicles contract closer to the body, and the pelvis, buttocks, and leg muscles tense. Muscles around the prostate gland squeeze out semen along the urethra, and sperm travels up and out through the vas deferens, resulting in ejaculation.

Genital armoring in men can be caused by attempts to conform with "macho" posturing and attitudes, unnecessarily rough prostate examinations, and fearful or guilty sexual experiences. Armoring can either block sexual excitement, resulting in a man having difficulty in achieving an erection, or may manifest as extreme tension in the lingam and muscles causing a need for intense stimulation to bring about orgasmic release.

Relaxing, aromatic baths and massage are especially important for men and help to diffuse sexual response throughout the body. Experiencing sex as a sensual process rather than a goal-oriented performance driving toward an orgasmic "touchdown" takes off the pressure that many men feel and that actually inhibits full sexual enjoyment. Most men respond favorably to the arousing aromas and grounding or relaxing properties of the following:

Lingam Essences

Bergamot	Bay laurel	Cedar	Cinnamon
Ginger	Jasmine	Patchouli	Rose
Sandalwood	Vanilla	Vetiver	Ylang-ylang

A Rose by Any Other Name:
Yoni and Lingam Love Names

WE MUST TURN TO THE EAST to find beautiful, evocative names for the sex organs, as our own language really provides none. We have technical terms, we have derogatory slang terms, but we have nothing to rival "The Gate of Jewels" (Japanese), "The Diamond Scepter" (Sanskrit), or "The Purple Mushroom Peak" (Chinese). Just for fun, here are lists of yoni and lingam names to increase your vocabulary of love.

Yoni Names

Cinnabar Cleft (Taoist)
Pure Lily (Chinese)
Mysterious Gateway (Taoist)
Doorway of Life (Chinese)
Secret Cavern (Chinese)
Mystic Rose (Western esoteric)
Inner Heart (Chinese)
The Lotus of Her Wisdom
  (Sanskrit)

Jade Gate (Chinese)
Concha (Latin)
Red Pearl (Chinese)
Mysterious Valley (Taoist)
Golden Gate (Chinese)
Sensitive Cave (Chinese)
Pillow of Musk (Chinese)

Lingam Names

Ambassador (Chinese)
Plough (Tantric)
Jade Scepter (Chinese)
Crimson Bird (Chinese)
Spear (Sanskrit)
Magic Wand (Western esoteric)
Discoverer (Arabic)

Jade Flute (Chinese)
Arrow of Love (Tantric)
Searcher (Arabic)
Key of Desire (Persian)
Dart (Arabic)
Yang Peak (Chinese)
Mushroom of Immortality
  (Chinese)

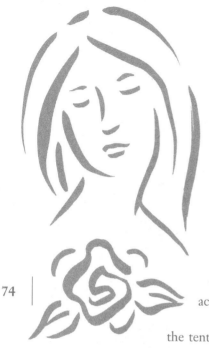

FEMALE HOT SPOTS

A kiss is the most potent aphrodisiac.

EUROPEAN SAYING

There's a good reason for that! According to the Tantric energy system, there are fourteen major and thousands of lesser *nadis* (Sanskrit for "vein" or "tube") crisscrossing the body, which carry subtle energies from one *chakra*, or energy center, to the next. This concept is similar to the Chinese idea of "meridians," invisible energy highways that can be strengthened or unblocked through the use of acupuncture and shiatsu.

The *shankhini nadi*, described by an ancient Tantric text as the tenth, secret opening of the body, runs from a woman's lips and palate down through the breast, creating a direct link to her yoni, and back up again. Stimulation of the mouth through kissing, and of the nipples through kissing and massage, sends a strong current of energy down to the clitoris, dramatically increasing sexual arousal. The stronger the energy flow along this nadi, the deeper and more intense a woman's level of arousal. To strengthen the shankhini nadi and increase your capacity for sexual excitement, try the following.

ESSCENTUAL EXERCISE:
STRENGTHENING THE SHANKHINI NADI

Begin by relaxing and taking a few deep breaths. Choose an essence from the list of the yoni essences. Rest the upper edge of the vial lightly against your upper lip as you inhale the aroma. This is the beginning point of the nadi. Feel the scent penetrating your palate, then moving along a bright skein of energy that plays through your skull, down the back of your neck, through the shoulder and heart, under your left nipple, behind your navel, and down into the clitoris or G-spot. Touch your finger lightly to your clitoris, and breathe deeply of the essence near your upper lip, feeling both ends of the nadi, and the increasing flow of energy between the two spots.

The next time you make love, try visualizing the energy flow along the nadi to enhance your sense of arousal. Your partner can help by stimulating the beginning of the nadi with gentle, probing kisses, then proceed to light, rolling massage of your nipples and breasts with a blend of massage oil and a few drops of yoni essences. Stimulation of the clitoris and G-spot completes and enhances the energy flow, and should have you well on your way to full sexual arousal.

INCREASING FEMALE SEXUAL RESPONSIVENESS:
THE PC PUMP AND G-SPOT MASSAGE

Female sexual responsiveness rises and falls in cycles. Desire for sexual contact increases after ovulation, peaking at a time just before or during menstruation. Just after menstruation, a woman's sexual appetite may be at its lowest ebb. Taking cyclical response into consideration can save a lot of puzzlement and frustration between lovers, who may otherwise be disappointed if a flood of sexual feeling fails to materialize at "low tide."

"PC" stands for "pubucoccygeus," the butterflylike muscle that connects the front of the pelvis to the lower spine and the anus and genitals to the sitting bones and legs. The yoni is supported all around by a figure eight of muscles that extend around the vagina, urethra, and anus. The PC is the largest of these muscles, which grip and massage the lingam during lovemaking and which contract involuntarily during female orgasm. Getting control of these muscles and keeping them strong contributes immensely to sexual enjoyment for both partners and helps to keep the vagina toned and healthy.

To do the "PC Pump," think of what it feels like when you need to urinate, but the bathroom is far away. This is the muscle you use to "hold it." Tighten the muscle as you inhale. Hold it for a count of ten. Then release as you exhale. Continue for as many repetitions as you can, starting with ten to twenty pumps a day and working up from there. Once the muscle is in shape, try doing the pump deliberately during lovemaking to increase your arousal and your partner's enjoyment.

G-Spot massage can be done alone or with a partner, to increase sensitivity in the yoni and to magnify sexual response. As with any developing ability, sexual responsiveness increases with positive experiences and plenty of practice! Start with a warm, relaxing bath utilizing a few drops of yoni essences, followed by a massage or body rub using oil into which yoni essences have been blended.

Gently begin to create a state of sexual arousal, using the nadi visualization. Stimulate and tickle the nipples and clitoris, stroke the belly, the buttocks, and the insides of the thighs. Lubricate the yoni if necessary, and when ready, introduce a finger slowly into the vagina. Explore carefully and gently the soft but firm and smooth area that begins just behind the rougher folds of the inner lips and hymen. Stroke with the fingertips (make sure nails are clipped short!) and explore until you find a spot that gives you a pleasurable, slightly electric sensation. As arousal progresses, you will feel the inside of the yoni growing softer, wetter, and more elastic, moving and changing shape as you approach orgasm. Allow your hips and legs to move rhythmically and freely, rising or circling in whatever way feels good to you. Breathe slowly and deeply into the pleasure, as the sensations spread through your body. Note what feels the best to you, where, and how, and if doing the exercise with a partner, say so! Stimulation of the G-Spot often culminates in an orgasm that can flow upwards through the entire body, or it may feel focused in a particular area, such as the lower spine, breasts, throat, or uterus.

Using an essential oil such as **ylang-ylang**, **jasmine**, **rose**, or **neroli** during this exercise provides additional relaxation and arousal. The essence can become associated with orgasmic sensations and be used on other sexual occasions to heighten response.

INCREASING MALE RESPONSIVENESS:
LINGAM MASSAGE

Releasing tensions that may be held in the musculature surrounding the lingam can increase a man's sexual pleasure and assist in diffusing erotic sensations beyond the area of the genitals, opening up possibilities for fuller, even whole-body orgasm. Alternate tension-relieving massage of the thighs and tissues surrounding the genitals with pleasurable stroking of the lingam and scrotum to create an experience for your lover that is both healing and enjoyable.

The ideal essence to use with this exercise is **sandalwood**, in a dilution of 5 to 10 drops of essence in half an ounce of carrier oil, such as sesame. **Rose** is a good choice too. Allow at least half an hour of uninterrupted time for the exercise.

The man relaxes back into a bank of pillows, on his back, with his legs comfortably apart. Make sure your hands, and the oil, are warm and that your nails are short, as the area you will be massaging is highly sensitive. Take a few deep breaths together before you begin, to relax and become present. The lover receiving the massage needs to focus his awareness within and to be able to remain quietly open to receive the healing touch of his partner. Any thoughts, feelings, or memories that surface can be shared at the time they occur, or later, whatever feels right.

Anoint the lingam and the area surrounding it liberally with oil. Ask your lover to breathe into the area as you work, gently exploring the muscles, tendons, and tissues. You may come across areas that are tender, or discover small, crystallized knots of tension. The idea is not to cause pain in these areas, but quietly to bring your lover's awareness to them. Massage gently, encouraging your lover to recall when he first remembers feeling pain or tension in that area. What was happening in his life at the time? Is it keyed to an experience or an event? Is your lover ready to release any pain or emotion that may be trapped there? If so, encourage him to breathe deeply through the experience, whether he is able to talk about it or not, to allow the trapped energies to dissolve and be released completely. If no clear memory comes to mind, let it be. It may be enough that the area has drawn attention to itself, and attracted your lover's conscious awareness. Healing and release will happen in their own perfect time.

The Scented Rainbow of Love:
Chakra Meditation

ECSTASY IS A FREE FLOW OF ENERGY, a sense of oneness and connectedness with each other and with all things. While there is always an invisible exchange of energy going on between lovers, the process is not always a conscious one. This meditation exercise facilitates the flow of life force through the chakras of the body, and uses the fragrances of essential oils and visualization to consciously connect your energy centers with the chakra energies of your lover.

Things can happen during this meditation! You may experience a heaviness, or block, at certain chakra levels, or you may be surprised by a sudden intensity of energy flow between the two of you. You may find levels at which you and your lover have difficulty connecting. Whatever happens, it's okay. Let the aromas of the essences waft through blocks or obstacles, to carry you easily from one level to the next. Relax, inwardly acknowledge your thoughts and feelings, and allow them to pass through you. Remember, this is a process of discovery. As with love, the journey is the destination.

To begin, purify the space in which you'll be meditating by smudging with sage or burning incense. Unplug the phone. It's best if, once you begin, you go through the exercise to the end without speaking or touching, and with no interruptions. Choose seven oils, one to correspond with each chakra, and set them up in the order that you'll be using them. Or, to make it even simpler, create a "Seven Chakra Blend" by blending essences that resonate with all seven chakras. You can blend the essences together in a vial, or mix them with a carrier oil and use a small amount to anoint the outside of the body in the area of each chakra as you go through the meditation.

Seven Chakra Blends

patchouli, jasmine, orange, bergamot, sandalwood, rose

ℰ

myrrh, vanilla, ginger, benzoin, cedar

ℰ

rosewood, bay laurel, clary sage, chamomile, helichrysm, lavender

ℰ

vetiver, sandalwood, black pepper, bergamot, jasmine, frankincense

ℰ

elemi, sandalwood, clary sage, rosemary, eucalyptus, balsam fir

ℰ

frankincense, rose, vetiver, benzoin

ℰ

oakmoss, jasmine, cedar, bergamot, ginger

To BEGIN, sit comfortably opposite your lover, the essences within easy reach of both of you. Scatter a circle of rose petals or fresh lovers' flowers around yourselves (see the list at the end of chapter 8). Dedicate your space, either silently or verbally, with an acknowledgment such as "Enclosed within this fragrant circle is a sacred space, bounded and protected by Love, and a place in which Love flows freely between us."

Take a few moments to center and relax, breathing deeply.

FIRST CHAKRA:
RED

Sexuality, Connecting with the Earth

Essential oils: patchouli, vetiver, oakmoss, tonka bean, rosewood, angelica, frankincense, myrrh, elemi (to link first and seventh chakras)

Focus on the base of the spine, or the perineum (the place between the genitals and the anus). This is the *muladhara*, the "root" or base chakra. This energy center connects you with the Earth, and is the source of the vital energy you need to take care of things basic to your own survival. It is also associated with your sense of smell. Imagine it as a point of deep, intense red that spreads out, disclike, through your body. Now reach for the essence you have chosen for this chakra. As you breathe in its aroma, visualize it going down through your body and being soaked up by the red disc. Pass the oil to your lover. Once both of you have inhaled its aroma, return the bottle to its place. Close your eyes, and imagine the fragrance shooting out in an arc of red light from both your root chakras, meeting at a midpoint in the space between you. Allow the aroma and the red light to mingle and connect the two of you at root chakra level. Take a few moments to experience and enjoy the connection. With a bit of practice, you'll know intuitively when the energy connection has been established and when it's time to move on to the next level.

SECOND CHAKRA:
ORANGE

Sexuality and Creativity

Essential Oils: ylang-ylang, vanilla, cardamom, jasmine and rose (also fourth and seventh chakras), **sandalwood** (also seventh)

Now focus on a spot about midway between pubis and navel. This is the *svadhishth ana*, the spleen or sacral chakra. This energy center is associated with sexuality, creativity, reproductive and hormonal processes, and the sense of taste. Think of it as bright orange-red. Choose your oil, allowing the fragrance to flow down through you, through the chakra, and out to connect with the energy of your partner. In your mind, visualize the flowing arc of orange as a second layer on the pulsating red that the two of you have already established.

THIRD CHAKRA:
YELLOW

Center of the Self, Inner Fire and Passion

Essential Oils: ginger, bay laurel, black pepper, orange, eucalyptus (also fifth), **juniper and vetiver** (protective and cleansing)

Next is the *manipura*, the navel or solar plexus chakra. This is an important energy center in many Eastern traditions. It corresponds to the middle *tan-t'ien*, or energy gate of Taoism, which is the source of *ch'i*, the vital spirit/breath and cosmic force that animates all life forms. Among the Sufis, it is considered to be the center of the self. The energy that moves you through the activities of the physical world is expressed through this chakra, which is located in the solar plexus, just above the belly button. It is also associated with joie de vivre, physical intuition (the "gut feeling"), physical magnetism, and the sense of sight. Imagine this chakra as glowing with radiant yellow light. Share the fragrance of the oil you have chosen with your lover, and visualize a yellow rainbow band above the orange and red already connecting you.

FOURTH CHAKRA:
GREEN/PINK

Love

Essential Oils: rose, jasmine, melissa, neroli, clary sage, lemon verbena, geranium, benzoin (also seventh)

The fourth chakra is the *anahata*, or heart chakra, located in the center of the chest in the area of the heart. Called the "secret center" among the Sufis, this chakra is associated with love and compassion and the sense of touch. In Taoism, the same area is called the "Heavenly Fire of the Heart." Whereas the first three energy centers are physically oriented, this one functions as an intermediary between the body and the mind, between the physical demands of existence and the subtler energies of the higher chakras.

For many people, this is a difficult chakra to keep open. Removing the armor we often build around this energy center requires the release of past trauma and pain and may leave us frighteningly vulnerable to additional hurts. Yet a free flow of energy from this center is crucial to being able to give and receive love. "Stay heart-wounded," as one spiritual teacher advises, meaning that we must have the courage to love even when we know that doing so will sometimes bring us pain. This is also what Christ meant by "turning the other cheek." Visualize this energy center as surrounded and intersected by a disc of clear green, with a center of warm and golden pink, blossoming from deep within your heart. I highly recommend using the aroma of rose with this chakra, the essence or absolute if you can get it, or a fresh flower (not an unscented variety). Rose is what love smells like, according to thousands of years of tradition! Let the green and pink energy you have visualized form another connective band of rainbow energy between you and your love.

FIFTH CHAKRA:
BLUE

Communication, Personal Expression

Essential Oils: blue chamomile, Roman chamomile, bergamot, tanacetum anum, eucalyptus, benzoin (also fourth and seventh)

The *vishuddha* (Sanskrit for "pure") chakra is located at the base of the throat, and is associated with creativity, communication, self-expression, and the sense of hearing. Anger and fear may block this chakra, resulting in a tight, strained voice and a restricted or "lumpy" feeling in the neck and throat. Words like "I love you" can get stuck in this energy center if it closes and may be difficult to say. Singing, growling, and chanting will help to open it up again. Visualize this chakra as bathed in blue. Share your essence with your lover, and imagine the shimmering blue, scented band that builds another, higher level of connection on your rainbow bridge.

SIXTH CHAKRA:
INDIGO

Opening Consciousness, Psychic Abilities and Intuition

Essential Oils: cedar, cistus, elemi, mugwort, helichrysm, rosemary, peppermint, fir, frankincense, sandalwood, and spruce (all also seventh)

Deep within the brain is *ajna*, the brow or "third eye" chakra. This is the seat of the synthesis of thought processes and the place of origin for psychic awareness. Imagine a two-petaled lotus of deep indigo opening inside your head. Choose your essence, and feel the fragrance form a loop as it enters your nostrils, passes through your brain, and floats out again through your forehead at a point just above and between your eyes, on a band of indigo light connecting you with your partner.

SEVENTH CHAKRA:
VIOLET OR WHITE (ALL COLORS)

Union of Souls, Connection with Cosmic Forces

Essential Oils: rose, jasmine, sandalwood, rosewood, lavender, frankincense, myrrh, benzoin, fir, spruce

Sahasrara, Sanskrit for thousand, describes the energy center at the crown, or top of the head, which is visualized as a thousand-petaled, rainbow-colored lotus. I never really understood why, until in the course of some spiritual work, this chakra was opened for me. It literally felt as if thousands of petals were opening and unfolding in the top of my skull. Among the Sufis, this center is known as "the teacher."

This energy center is associated with the integration of all levels of being into a harmonious and liberated whole. It is also the gateway to cosmic consciousness. Imagine the top of your head bathed in violet, shooting forth rainbows of light. Choose your seventh essence, and allow the fragrance to mingle with the shooting rainbows as they dance toward union with your lover.

Visualize now the free flow of rainbow energy between you and your lover as a wheel of fragrance, light, and color turning clockwise. It flows into one of you, through the other, and back again, ever-moving, ever-changing, ever there. Breathe deeply, becoming aware of the mingled aromas of the essences as they escape in tendrils of scent from their open bottles, volatilizing in the air, riding in on your breath, passing through you as Life and Love pass through you. The fragrances are just another movement of energy, pure Being in another of its many disguises.

There is no beginning to the flow of energy now, and there is no end. Allow it to move freely between the two of you for a few moments, then slowly center within yourself. Cap your oils, inwardly acknowledging your appreciation for anything they may have shown to you or revealed in the course of the exercise. End the meditation with a kiss to your lover and a warm embrace.

As this becomes an easy and fluid exercise for you and your partner, you may want to add one more energy center to your meditation.

EIGHTH CHAKRA:
SILVER/GOLD

Spiritual Purpose, Angelic Guidance

Essential Oils: frankincense, rose (steam distilled), **lavender, neroli**

Above the head, located in the invisible energy field that surrounds your physical body, is an eighth chakra, representative of your highest aspirations and mission in life. As you meditate on this energy center, realize that part of being human is to exist as a bridge between heaven and earth. It's not always easy to keep it all in balance. To the soul is given the demanding task of filtering day-to-day experience, transmuting earthly energies, and transforming reality with love. Invite angelic guidance to help clarify your path, when you and your lover are ready to attune yourselves and your relationship to resonate with the will of the Divine.

SEVEN

The Esscentual Experience:
A Night of Love

Once the wheel of Love has been set in motion,
there is no absolute rule.

KAMA SUTRA

WHETHER YOU'RE PLANNING AN AROMATIC INTERLUDE with a brand-new lover or a longtime flame, don't make the mistake of waiting until you get into bed for the foreplay to begin. Start early by appealing to that most powerful of all human erogenous zones, the brain. Get your lover thinking about you and fantasizing about the esscentual delights you have in store. Make quick, suggestive phone calls; tuck love notes into a pocket, purse, or car, scented with aphrodisiac essences (especially blends your lover will recognize, such as those you've previously used together with amorous success). An unexpected gift of flowers or a custom-blended massage oil or perfume can get the romantic imagination rolling. If you're married or

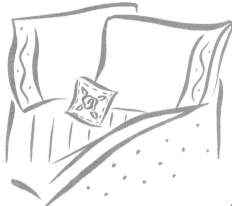

living together, you can leave esscentual clues along your lover's well-worn daily path to signal that something special is about to happen . . . soon.

Prepare as much as you can in advance, leaving plenty of room for spontaneity and the unexpected. Make up your blends beforehand and have them easily accessible, along with clean towels, erotic books or toys, robes, candles, musical selections, or anything else you might conceivably need. Give the room a thorough once-over, making certain that everything is pleasantly clean. Rinse sheets and bedclothes in aromatic floral waters, or include a few drops of an aphrodisiac essence in the final rinse or on a cloth thrown in for the last few minutes of drying.

The once-over should also include cleansing the vibration of the room, so that the energy within is peaceful and calm. Smudge sticks or incense of sage, cedar, or juniper lift the atmosphere, and any heavy or unpleasant energy residue is carried away on the fragrant smoke. Smudge sticks, traditionally used by Native Americans as part of purification ceremonies, are fairly easy to find at health food stores and new age bookshops, or you can make your own from bunches of dried herbs wrapped securely with thread. (A recipe for incense is included in the next chapter.) Allow the smoke to penetrate all the nooks and crannies, paying especial attention to corners and closets. Visualize the room filling with light and the warm, positive energy of love. You could also fill a sprayer bottle with water and add a few drops of **juniper**, **cedar**, or **angelica** essential oil, then spritz all round, to get the same effect.

Think in advance about what you're going to eat and drink. A recent study comparing famous love scenes in literature turned up the amazing observation that every single one of them was preceded by some kind of erotic repast. It doesn't have to be a wild and sloppy orgiastic eating experience like in the movie classic *Tom Jones*, or an all-out multicourse production number like *Babette's Feast*. But eating together definitely raises erotic sensibilities, especially when aromatic aphrodisiac elements are incorporated into the menu, such as in the recipes that are included in the next chapter to get you started.

Plan to spend an evening, a night, and a morning together. Unplug the phone and the TV. Savor each moment as you celebrate the miracle of loving and simply being together. Just for tonight, you are devoted only to the esscentual delights you can create for each other. All your responsibilities, duties, and ceaseless activities will still be there tomorrow. For tonight, how much pleasure can you arouse in your lover? Is there a limit to the passion you can experience together? How high can you take each other? How deeply can you love?

Following are two esscentual experiences you and your lover can try, based on information presented in the book. Feel free to improvise, or to start from scratch and create your own magic using the aromatic knowledge you've been given. Candles, incense, potpourris, and diffusers create an erotic aura through environmental fragrancing. Aromatic baths are very esscentual, and leave you warm, clean, and fragrant for amorous play. Perfume and massage oils enhance arousal through touch. Fragrant flowers are visually beautiful and send a subtle sexual message. Once considered to be both the food and the aroma of gods and goddesses, Nature's precious essences nourish the heart and enhance intimacy by penetrating to the core of love.

Shiva and Shakti

DELIGHT YOUR LOVER with this esscentual evocation of erotic response, inspired by an ancient Tantric ritual. Prepare your bedroom or space with careful attention to texture and color. Violet, the Tantric color of female sexual energy, and red, the color of vitality and life force, should dominate. Silk, velvet, satin, fur, and feathers are all interesting textures for you and your lover to play with. Create small piles of symbolic yoni and lingam objects, to honor your sexuality and for visual and subconscious appeal. (Yoni symbols include shells, triangles, almonds, eggs, horseshoes, fresh apricots, and flowers. Lingam symbols are crystals, wands, and bananas.)

Signal the beginning of the experience with a musical sound, such as a triangle, gong, Tibetan bell, or singing bowl. Relax into the space with a glass of wine or other aphrodisiac beverage, such as Armagnac, cognac, Metaxa, Benedictine, Chartreuse, or coconut milk mixed with honey. You might also want to indulge in some aphrodisiac snacks, such as chocolate, truffles, oysters, pomegranates, coconut, or pumpkin seeds. If you have erotic art or Tantric pillowbooks, quietly contemplate them together as you feel your desires rise.

You will be using aromatherapy essences as Tantric perfumes to anoint the marmas, or erogenous zones, of your partner. These zones are basically the same in both male and female, and you can do them all on one lover from beginning to end, or alternate between the two of you. Relax, take your time, and enjoy. The idea is to create an erotic symphony of scent, touch, taste, vision, and sound. Make sexy noises. Tune into each other. Turn each other on. Tell each other which aromas you like the best. Don't be afraid to laugh!

The anointing begins with the Secondary Marmas. Put a drop or two of **rose**, **geranium**, or **spikenard** on your fingertips and run them through your lover's hair, pausing to gently caress the earlobes, then the nape of the neck.

Have your lover lean back comfortably on a mound of pillows. Using a diluted blend of **sandalwood** (5 drops to a half ounce of oil), massage the base of the spine and the insides of the thighs, gradually shifting focus to stimulating the lingam or yoni, the first of the Primary Marmas. Erection and penetration are not the point here. The partner being anointed simply accepts the pleasure.

Move on to massaging the breasts and nipples with **patchouli** (in similar dilution), and use the same oil to anoint the cheeks. Stimulate the lip/tongue marma with deep and sensual kissing. Then anoint the palms of the receptive lover's hands with a dilution of **jasmine**, including the wrists and fingers in your massage of this Tertiary Marma. **Saffron** or **rose** is used on the soles of the feet. Other Tertiary Marmas include the apertures of the ears, the navel, and the front insides of the nostrils.

Once you've awakened all the senses and pleasure centers of your bodies, be spontaneous. Let your bodies resonate with the giving and receiving of erotic energy. Rub your scented parts against each other, mixing and mingling all the various fragrances. The aromas will change subtly with friction, warmth, and the passage of time. Continue to anoint each other, wherever and however you are inspired to do so. Let your lovemaking create a unique and beautiful perfume!

Antony and Cleopatra

TO CREATE A ROMANTIC EGYPTIAN EVENING for your lover, use a few choice weapons from Cleopatra's scentual arsenal. Rinse your robes, lingerie, and/or bedsheets in Bulgarian **rose water**, letting them air-dry to preserve the delicate fragrance. Scent your hair with **jasmine**, putting a drop or two on your brush, then brushing until your hair is fragrant and shiny. Burn kyphi incense (see recipe, next chapter) in the bedroom before your lover arrives to create an exotic atmosphere. Scatter mounds of fresh red rose petals on the bedside table, and tuck some into your pillows. (You can put a few on the bed for visual effect, but too many will have an unromantic way of sticking to the skin.) Float fresh, fragrant flowers such as gardenia, lotus, or full-blown roses in bowls of water. (Antony and Cleopatra would string garlands of fresh, fragrant flowers and put them around each other's necks. They floated smaller blossoms in their wine glasses.) Have a basket of luscious fresh figs within easy reach, as a before- or after-love snack. (But please, leave out the asp!)

℮

These are only two possible ways of using aromatherapy for lovers to create an esscentual experience. Use your imagination to come up with more! The possibilities are truly endless. All you really need are a few carefully chosen oils, a lover, some time, and a healthy and creative sense of play!

Morning Transitions

THE MORNING AFTER THE NIGHT BEFORE can be an especially delicate time for lovers. It's not always easy to make the transition from the passions of the night to the scheduled duties and rigors of the day. Lovers may feel awkward with each other, vulnerable or emotionally exposed. The person you were so freely intimate with under cover of candles and darkness may suddenly seem like a stranger in the gathering light of dawn.

Be prepared! Have a few comforting, confidence-enhancing, or morning pick-me-up essences on hand to smooth the transition into the day. Essences can be diffused throughout the house or apartment to wake up the senses, or blended into stimulating shower gels and shampoos. Floral waters or water with a few drops of essence added can be kept in a sprayer bottle, shaken up and spritzed on face and body to awaken and refresh.

The other precaution you need to take is not to overschedule yourself. Allow plenty of time for a leisurely morning. You don't want to have to jump out of bed and run out the door, or rush a new lover through a quick shower and breakfast on the run.

Morning Pick-Me-Ups

Grapefruit	Lemon	Nutmeg	Black pepper
Tangerine	Rosemary	Coriander	Lemongrass
Orange	Peppermint	Balsam fir	Basil

Confidence Enhancers

Bay laurel	Sandalwood	Clary sage	Jasmine
Lime	Lavender	Ginger	Chamomile
Cedar	Geranium	Clove	Turkish rose

Once you're alert and awake, take a few minutes to share breakfast with your lover before going your separate ways. (I highly recommend the Rose Petal Love Scones in chapter 9!) Consider the morning after when you plan your esscentual experience, and it can be the happy ending note (or coda!) to a joyful night of love-making and the prelude to many beautiful shared experiences to come.

EIGHT

A Complete Listing of
Aphrodisiac Essential Oils and Absolutes

FOLLOWING IS A LISTING OF ESSENTIAL OILS, followed by their botanical names and a brief description, which includes some history and the skin/hair type the fragrance of the essence is thought to suit best. This doesn't mean that if you're blond, for example, you should never use ambrette because it's recommended for the red-haired male. It only means that the oil has been used traditionally to complement that particular type. It gives you a bit of a head start, especially when blending for someone else. For personal use, you'll want to experiment with each of the oils to discover what smells best, both to you and on you.

AMBRETTE *Hibiscus moschata*
Aroma: Warm, animal

Made from hibiscus seeds, ambrette has a musk-like scent and is often used in aromatherapy perfume blending as a musk substitute. The essence contains farnesol, a bacteriostatic and skin-soothing constituent that is also present in rose. Hindu brides were traditionally anointed with a perfume oil made of ambrette and jasmine on their wedding night. A favorite perfume in China and Japan. Especially compatible with the fair, red-haired male.

ANGELICA *Angelica archangelica*
Aroma: Earthy, animal

Another musk substitute, distilled from seeds or roots. The seed essence is fresh, light, peppery; more common is the root essence, earthy and herbal smelling, with animal undertones. Used to flavor the liqueurs Cointreau and Chartreuse. Kills microorganisms that cause yellow fever (as do essences of cinnamon, thyme, and sandalwood). Especially compatible with the fair, red-haired female.

BASIL *Ocimum basilicum*
Aroma: Herbal, aromatic, stimulating

Basil gets its name from the Greek word for "king," basileus. Tulsi, the holy basil of India, is sacred to Krishna and Vishnu, planted around Hindu temples, and included in a fragrant oil used daily by Indian kings (for the recipe, see chapter 9). Stimulates the sympathetic nervous system and overall male sexual response. In Italy, the country name for basil translates as "Kiss Me, Nicholas," and is synonymous with love. In Northern Europe, a girl's virginity was put to the test by having her walk through a swarm of bees holding basil in her hands. (If she was stung, or if the leaves withered, she was considered unchaste.) Especially compatible with dark-haired men.

BAY LAUREL *Laurus nobilis*
Aroma: Strong, spicy

In ancient Rome, this herb crowned the victor. Its name comes from the Latin *laudare*, to praise. "Bay" is from an Anglo-Saxon word meaning chaplet, or crown, and gave rise to the expression "keeping at bay," because the herb's aroma was believed to counteract plague. Laurel was also used by Roman warriors in baths to comfort aching limbs and fatigued senses after battle and as a strewing herb among Elizabethans. A confidence boosting, "first date" kind of essence, or great for a nervous groom on his wedding day! Especially compatible with the dark-haired male.

BENZOIN *Styrax benzoin* (Sumatra), *S. tonkinense* (Indochina)
also known as gum benzoin, gum benjamin
Aroma: Sweet, balsamic, vanilla-like

Used in the form of an alcohol tincture in aromatherapy, this resin is collected from the wounded bark of balsam trees that are at least six years old and are grown in the forests of India, Java, Sumatra, Cambodia, and Thailand. The name is a corruption of the Arabic, *luban jawi*, meaning "incense of Java," as it was once considered another form of frankincense (which was also known as *luban*). Arabs originally bought it from the Hindus and sold it to the Chinese spice market and European buyers, all of whom used it medicinally and for fragrance. The Malays used it to ward off devils, and the gum resin is burned in India before the sacred Trimurti, the combined faces of Brahma, Shiva, and Vishnu. Especially compatible with blond men and women.

BERGAMOT *Citrus bergamia*
Aroma: Fresh, a bit fruity

This greenish-tinted essence is expressed from the peel of the Bergamo orange and is an important ingredient in real *eau de cologne* and perfumery in general. Its unique fragrance is due to an ester, linalyl acetate, which is also a chief constituent of lavender oil. Especially compatible with brown-haired men and women. **Caution: Do not use on skin before exposure to sun, as permanent pigment discoloration can result.** (This problem is eliminated if you can find an essence of bergamot which does not contain bergaptene. If you're not sure, don't take a chance.)

BLACK PEPPER *Piper nigrum*
Aroma: Light, peppery, warming

Long considered an aphrodisiac among the Arabs, who boiled eggs with black pepper, cinnamon, and myrrh as a libido-stimulating dish. The essence is effective for warming and stimulating men in general, especially the freckled, red-haired kind. **Caution: Use sparingly, as spice oils can be irritating to the skin.**

CARDAMOM *Elletaria cardamomum*
Aroma: Fresh, spicy

Distilled from the seeds, a high-quality oil has a beautiful, light spiciness; the cheaper grades can smell harsh and medicinal. After saffron, this is the world's most expensive spice and has been used for thousands of years. First mentioned in 4th century B.C. Ayurvedic medical texts, the spice has been exported since Hellenistic times. Used extensively in India as an aphrodisiac. An Arab aphrodisiac dish blends powdered cardamom, ginger, and cinnamon sprinkled over boiled onions. Especially effective for the red-haired male. **Caution: Use sparingly, as spice oils can be irritating to the skin.**

CARNATION *Dianthus caryophyllus*
Aroma: Heavy, sweet, honey-like

This is a rare and costly absolute, used more in perfumery than in practical aromatherapy. In her excellent book *Aromantics*, Valerie Worwood suggests that a blend of ylang-ylang and pepper can create a plausible fragrance imitation of the fresh flower's peppery aroma. Carnation absolute is a confidence-building aroma that helps create a strong inner sense of self, one of the vital ingredients for physical magnetism and attractiveness. Especially effective for brown-haired women and men.

CEDAR *Cedrus atlantica*
Aroma: Full, woody

In Mesopotamia, the cradle of civilization, cedar of Lebanon was used for healing, in exorcisms, and ritually after sex. It was also used in Babylonia, where its fragrance fed the ancestors and repelled bad spirits. Egyptians used cedarwood oil after bathing and started importing it in the year 2700 B.C. from Tyre. Cedar of Lebanon is now endangered and is no longer distilled. Instead, *C. atlantica*, from Morocco, is cut, chipped, and steam distilled. Especially suitable for the dark-haired male.

CHAMOMILE *Anthemis nobilis, Matricaria chamomilla*
Aroma: Sweet, herbal, fruity

An emotionally stabilizing oil distilled from flowers and stems and used in many cultures since ancient times by women and children in particular. It's also used as a flavoring for D.O.M. and Benedictine liqueurs. *A. nobilis* is known as "Roman" chamomile, *M. chamomilla* as "German" or "blue." The perfect oil for sensitive natures and sensitive skins and especially suited to blond women.

CHAMPAC *Michelia champaca*
Aroma: Heavy, sweet, floral

This rare and beloved essence from India can sometimes be found as an absolute or as an attar. Its velvety scent, reminiscent of ylang-ylang, blends well with rose, carnation, and sandalwood. Close relative of garden magnolias. Brought to China from India by Buddhist monks during the T'ang dynasty (7th–8th century). A scent especially for dark-haired men and women.

CINNAMON *Cinnamomum zeylanicum*
Aroma: Warm, spicy

This spice essence, revered since ancient times for its aphrodisiac qualities, is also highly antiseptic and antibacterial and has been shown to kill the typhoid bacillus within fifteen minutes. Cinnamon was an ingredient in Carmelite Water, which was said to have restored the failing powers of King Charles V of France in the 14th century. Especially compatible with the brown-haired male. **Caution: Use sparingly, as all spice oils can be irritating to the skin.**

CISTUS *Cistus ladaniferum* also known as "Labdanum" or Rockrose
Aroma: Sweet, honey-like, musky

Like myrrh, cistus was used as a base for many ancient perfumes, due to its narcotic aroma. Native to Crete, Greece, Macedonia, Syria, and Palestine, the viscous resin was exuded by bushes and collected by shepherds and goatherds who combed it from their animals' fleece. The French oil is finer in fragrance and lighter in color than that of North Africa or Spain. A good substitute for musk. Especially compatible with brown-haired men and women.

CLARY SAGE *Salvia sclarea*
Aroma: Heavy, herbal, musky

This wonderful euphoric and relaxant is a good friend to a woman's sexual response, especially when she's feeling inhibited due to tension and stress. Once used to flavor and intensify the intoxicating power of muscatel wine, clary sage is also important in perfumery, where it is the closest substitute to the animal fixative ambergris. Clary sage is closely related to garden sage, which Hippocrates recommended as a postwar tea for women to increase overall fertility. Especially effective with brown-haired men and women. **Caution: Do not use in conjunction with alcoholic beverages.**

CLOVE *Eugenia caryophyllata*
Aroma: Sweet, spicy, aromatic

Clove essence is distilled from the unopened buds and leaves of trees that may bear for a hundred years or more. Native to the Molucca Islands, clove is a powerful germ killer. One of its principal constituents, eugenol, is familiar to many as the smell of the dentist's office, as clove has been used traditionally for toothaches and dental hygiene. The fragrance of the distilled essence adds richness to rose and sweet floral blends. Especially recommended for dark-haired women, brown and dark-haired men. **Caution: Use sparingly and only in dilution, as it may cause skin irritation.**

CORIANDER *Coriandrum sativum*
Aroma: Spicy, sweet, woody

Coriander seeds, used by the ancient Egyptians for their stimulating and digestion-enhancing properties, have been found in tombs among the necessities that accompanied the deceased into the afterlife. It was mentioned as an aphrodisiac in *The*

Arabian Nights. The spice was called "dizzy corn" in medieval times, due to its slightly narcotic effect when too much was consumed, and was therefore used by boys who wanted to take advantage of country girls. The essential oil is used to flavor Chartreuse and Benedictine and in perfumery. Similar to cumin. A good scent for men in general.

COSTUS *Saussurea lappa*
Aroma: Green, with animal undertones

Known in India as "koosht," costus is made from the roots of a plant in the daisy and chrysanthemum family and is exported to China and Iran, where it is used to increase sexual activity. Kashmiri shawl makers tuck in costus, like patchouli, to keep insects away. It was once ground for use as incense. The extracted oil is very viscous, with a scent that has been variously described as orris root-like or resembling dirty hair.

CUMIN *Cuminum cyminum*
Aroma: Green, bitter, anise-like

Once used by Egyptian women during sex to ensure conception, cumin's properties are similar to those of coriander. It is a tonic and a stimulant to the heart and nervous system. One of the main ingredients of curry powder.

FENNEL *Foeniculum vulgare*
Aroma: Herbal, licorice-like

Fennel is another woman-friendly essence. The herb has been used for thousands of years to normalize body weight and to help balance the female reproductive system. It's also a good oil to use in baths and massage oils in conjunction with juniper, rosemary, cypress, lemon, or grapefruit to help ease water retention due to cellulitis or PMS. Especially compatible with blond females. **Caution: Fennel should not be used by children or epileptics.**

FRANKINCENSE *Boswellia serrata, B. carteri, B. thurifera*
also known as "Oil of Olibanum"
Aroma: Resinous, incense-like, exotic

From Isis to Aphrodite, from the temple of Baal and the Eleusinian mysteries to the Catholic church today, frankincense has played an important part in religious worship and is one of the most honored aromatic substances. From the same family as myrrh, its narcotic components open mind and spirit, expanding consciousness and breath. Especially compatible with the brown-haired male.

GERANIUM, ROSE *Pelargonium graveolens*

Aroma: Sweet, floral, rose-like

The presence of geraniol and phenyl ethyl alcohol, also important constituents of rose oil, explain the aromatic similarity and the use of less-expensive geranium to stretch the more precious essence of rose. Zdravets (*Geranium macrorhizum*), an exotic variety grown in Bulgaria, has a lively odor reminiscent of clary sage. Geranium stimulates the adrenal cortex, which influences levels of sex-related hormones in both men and women. Particularly suited to brown-haired males and females.

GINGER *Zingiber officinale*
Aroma: Warm, pungent, sweet/spicy

Women in Senegal pound ginger to wear in belts to stir their husbands' sexual interest, and both root and extracted oil have a fiery, warming effect. Closely related to cardamom, the essence blends well with citruses. Goes well with the red-haired man.

HYACINTH *Hyacinthus orientalis*
Aroma: Sweet, floral

Crowns of hyacinths were worn by maidens in attendance at ancient Greek weddings. This rare and costly absolute has a heady, intoxicating fragrance that especially suits red-haired women.

JASMINUM *officinale, J. grandiflorum, J. sambac*
Aroma: Seductive, sweet, floral

The sexiest flower fragrance on Earth. *J. officinale*, native to India, was the tip of one of the love god Kama's five arrows, which he used to pierce the heart through the senses. *J. grandiflorum* is more common in Europe. *J. sambac* is used in India for perfume and in China for tea. Jasmine is also grown in Grasse and was first cultivated in France in 1548, the result of trade with Arabs. Another important jasmine-growing area is Egypt, where it's handpicked by schoolchildren at dawn, before they go to school. The blossom breathes its most potent perfumes at dawn, and according to author Roy Genders, the aroma of white jasmine "can transform a woman into a nymphomaniac." Hindu poets call it "Moonlight of the Grove." Jasmine is found in almost all perfumes, including Eau Sauvage and Magie Noir (which also contain patchouli). An oil for every woman, and most men are fond of it too.

JUNIPER *Juniperus communis*
Aroma: Fresh, piney

Juniper has been used since ancient times as a sacred incense and to purify and protect physically, emotionally, and spiritually. The essential oil is distilled from the crushed berries, or sometimes from needles and branches. Spoons and forks were once made of the wood, to improve the taste of food, and clothes were kept fresh in juniper boxes. I include it here not for its aphrodisiac properties, which, as a general tonic, it might be presumed to have to some degree, but as a purifying oil for lovers to use when negative energies or emotions threaten to damage or destroy love. Juniper is the oil to use to clear the mind and body, and the air, after an argument or trauma.

LAVENDER *Lavandula officinalis, L. angustifolia*
Aroma: Fresh, sweet to camphorous

There are so many varieties of lavender, with accompanying variations of fragrance and effect, that they are too numerous to list here. The best lavender comes from France, and there's now a rare and beautiful essence available from the highlands of Bulgaria. English lavender is grown at Mitcham in Surrey, but is not available for export. Lavender is not a sexy oil per se, but it is a loving essence, due to its calming, soothing, and balancing qualities. Almost all men and women respond to its clean scent, which is said to be especially compatible with the red-haired female.

LIME *Citrus aurantiifolia*
Aroma: Green citrus, refreshing

Lime is a stimulating, refreshing essence that banishes depression and anxiety and is especially helpful in hot, muggy weather. Unlike other citrus oils, lime may be steam distilled or cold pressed. An important ingredient in colas. Recommended for dark-haired men and women.

MANDARIN *Citrus reticulata*
Aroma: Sweet, citrus

Once a gift to the mandarins of China, this sweet, calming essence pressed from the rind of the mandarin orange brings harmony and peace to fragile, sensitive spirits and combines beautifully with neroli and petitgrain for a synergistic effect of deep, sedative relaxation. Recommended for the fair, red-haired female.

MARJORAM *Origanum vulgare*
Aroma: Warm, herbal/spicy

Historical uses of marjoram associate it with both love and antiaphrodisiac effects. In aromatherapy the essence is considered the latter and is included here for its ability to appease the emotions and dissolve emotional tension. This is an oil to use when you need to cushion and mend during separations and endings, or to take a break from the intensity of a passionate relationship. **Caution: Overuse can have a dulling effect on the emotions.**

MELISSA *Melissa officinalis*
Aroma: Light, sweet, lemony

True melissa is as expensive as rose, and even more difficult to find. Melissa brings a sunshiny glow to body, mind, and spirit and is used in aromatherapy to balance the female reproductive system. Especially for the red-haired female. **Caution: Can be irritating and should be used in extreme dilution.**

MYRRH *Commiphora myrrha*
Aroma: Smoky, bitter

Myrrh is likely the oldest perfume used by human beings. Women of the East wore myrrh in small bags between their breasts, where the heat of their bodies released its aroma. The resin is taken from a prickly shrub that is native to Arabia, near the site of the Garden of Eden, which subsequently became the center of civilization and the perfume trade. In 1000 B.C. the Queen of Sheba brought myrrh seeds to Solomon to win his cooperation in allowing her to use incense trade routes that crossed his lands. The scent of myrrh is said to numb the senses when inhaled. The gum resin has a narcotic effect when immersed in wine, and was given by compassionate Jewesses to those about to be crucified during the Roman occupation of Israel. Praised in the Song of Songs and mentioned extensively in the tales of the Arabian Nights, myrrh is considered an aphrodisiac throughout the East. A Turkish aphrodisiac perfume blends frankincense, musk, and myrrh. Especially compatible with dark-haired men. **Caution: The essential oil should not be used by pregnant women.**

MYRTLE *Myrtis communis*
Aroma: Fresh, piney, crisp

In Babylon, myrtle was sacred to Shamash, the primordial god of the sun. Beloved in ancient Persian and Islamic gardens, myrtle was said by Muhammad to have fallen out of Paradise with Adam, clutched in his hand. Used in ancient times as a wedding decoration because of its association with Aphrodite, the evergreen plant was also awarded to poets by Greeks and Romans. The 1st-century Greek physician Rufus derived physiological names for the lips of the yoni from myrtle, the leaves of which he thought they resembled. Queen Esther took her name, Hadassah, from *hadas*, the Hebrew word for the shrub. Especially for blond females.

NARCISSUS *Narcissus poeticus*
Aroma: Heavy, sweet, narcotic

Narcissus is named for a handsome Greek who fell in love with his own reflection when he saw it in a pool of water. It was also the hypnotic fragrance of the flower that lured Persephone, daughter of the grain goddess Demeter, close enough to the shadows for Pluto, god of the underworld, to kidnap her, which he considered a perfectly acceptable way of obtaining a wife. Narcissus is rare, but occasionally available as an absolute.

NEROLI *Citrus aurantium*
Aroma: Rich, heady floral

The seductively scented essence of the blossom of the bitter orange was first brought to Italy from the East Indies by Portuguese sailors in the 12th century. It was given the name "neroli" centuries later, in honor of Anne Marie de la Tremoille-Noirmoutier, the Princesa Neroli, who was the second wife of wealthy 16th-century Roman aristocrat Flavio Orsini. Orange blossom was customarily part of wedding bouquets, due to its simultaneously sedative and seductive aromatic effect. An important ingredient in the popular perfume Poison. Recommended for blond women.

NUTMEG *Myristica fragrans*
Aroma: Warm, lightly spicy

Another of the many exotic and fragrant plants native to India, nutmeg was the aphrodisiac of choice among Chinese women. The essence is distilled by steam or carbon dioxide extraction from the seeds. Components of the essential oil iso-safrole and myrisiticine served as chemical blueprints for illicit drugs such as MDA and MMDA (also known as "ecstasy"). Especially for the red-haired female.

OAKMOSS *Evernia prunastri*
Aroma: Soft, powdery, honey-like

Used as a fixative in perfumes since pharaonic times, oakmoss is obtained by solvent extraction from a lichen that is native to the island of Cyprus, which is why it was included as an ingredient in the perfume *chypre*. The full, soft scent makes an excellent base for jasmine and blends beautifully with sandalwood.

ORRIS ROOT *Iris germanic, var. florentina; I. pallida*
Aroma: Sweet, violet-like

Rhizomes from the iris are dried for two to three years, then distilled or solvent extracted to make this very expensive, aphrodisiac essence. Powdered orris root is also available and is widely used as a fixative in fine potpourris. Orris root powder was also used extensively in Europe for hundreds of years to perfume wigs, sheets, and clothing.

PALMAROSA *Cymbopogon martini*
Aroma: Light, sweet, rosy

The sweet, floral-rosy aroma of a good palmarosa essence is due to its geraniol content, which makes it, like geranium, a popular way of stretching rose in a blend. Another native of India, the essence is distilled close to the fields where it is grown from stems, leaves, and flowering tops. Palmarosa is uplifting; it dispels dark clouds of anxiety and helps to bring peace of mind. The essence is also used in aromatherapy for skin care. Especially for dark-haired men.

PATCHOULI *Pogostemon cablin*, *P. heyneanus*, *P. patchouli*
Aroma: Earthy

Long known for its aphrodisiac qualities, patchouli is one of the most popular Tantric perfumes and an important ingredient in male and female perfumes such as Tabu, Aramis, Polo, Miss Dior, and Bill Blass. The essence is distilled from the leaves and stems of a soft-wooded shrub, a tropical member of the mint family, and gets its name from a Tamil word, *paccilai*, or green leaf. Good patchouli, such as that which is occasionally available from Egypt or India, will have a winelike sweetness. Generally, however, it is not a pretty smell but is lingering and stimulating to the senses. Especially for dark-haired women, red-haired males.

PEPPERMINT *Mentha piperita*
Aroma: Cool, penetrating, minty

Persephone, who was lured to the underworld with the scent of the narcissus, apparently got quite attached to her abductor and, in a fit of jealousy, turned the nymph Minta into this plant when she caught her messing around with Pluto. The herb, which combines "the coldness of betrayal with the heat of passion," has been cultivated and distilled in the United States since the nineteenth century and is used extensively for flavor and fragrance. An 1879 article in the *Lancet* brought about an explosion in its popularity by touting the medicinal benefits of menthol, the primary chemical constituent of peppermint oil, for relieving headaches and neuralgia. Though not an aphrodisiac per se, I include it here for its stimulating and healthful properties. **Caution: Use sparingly. May disrupt sleep if used late at night.** Also said to neutralize the effects of homeopathics.

PERU BALSAM *Myroxylon balsamum*, var. *pereirae*
Aroma: Rich, soft, sweet

Actually a native of El Salvador, this balsamic fixative is another resinous bark exudation, closely related to Balsam of Tolu (*Myroxylon balsamum*). Its rich and tenacious odor is due to the presence of cinnamic alcohol. Blends well with florals and spices.

PETITGRAINE *Petigrain bigarade*
Aroma: Fresh, floral

Chemically similar to neroli, this essence is distilled from the leaves of the bitter orange tree, whereas neroli is distilled from the blossoms. A good uplifting essence to blend with neroli to lessen some of the sedative effect and bring up the aphrodisiac qualities. Recommended for dark-haired females.

PINE *Pinus sylvestris*
Aroma: Clean, strong, piney

Distilled from the needles, pine is stimulating and invigorating, lending a sense of rootedness to the inner self. Used as a fragrance oil in ancient Egypt. Especially for blond men. **Caution: Use sparingly, as the undiluted essence can cause skin irritation.**

ROSE *Rosa damascena, R. centifolia*

If jasmine is the sexiest smell on earth, rose is the most beloved. (That's why I've honored it with its own chapter.) Sacred to Aurora, Venus, and the Virgin Mary, rose has been in common use for thousands of years as a symbol of love, joy, desire, beauty, femininity, and the divine. Valuable for increasing the sexual responsiveness of both men and women, aiding frigidity and impotence alike. Bulgarian rose is a fragrance for all women. The British aromatherapist Valerie Worwood recommends Rose Maroc as especially suited for redheads and black-haired women, and Turkish Rose as being better for blond and brunette women.

ROSEMARY *Rosmarinus officinalis*
Aroma: Clean, aromatic, herbal

Borneol acetate, a constituent also present in conifer oils, is what gives rosemary its invigorating aroma. One of the first ingredients used in alcohol perfumes, such as Hungary Water and Farina's original eau de cologne. A cephalic, or brain-stimulating oil, rosemary has been associated since ancient times with love and remembrance. Recommended for dark-haired women.

ROSEWOOD *Aniba rosaeodora*,
also known as Bois de rose
Aroma: Sweet, woody

It's a shame this essence is distilled from the wood of a rain forest tree that is on the verge of becoming an endangered species, because the aroma is so beautiful. A gentle, emotional aphrodisiac that clarifies romantic vision and promotes tranquillity. Especially for blond men.

SANDALWOOD *Santalum album*
Aroma: Honeyed wood

Called *chandana* in Sanskrit, sandalwood has been in continuous use for thousands of years and is the primary aromatic cultivated in India, where its availability is carefully guarded by the government. A semiparasitic tree, the sandalwood grows to thirty feet high and doesn't produce the essential oil in its heartwood until after thirty years of age. The aroma of sandalwood is centering and spiritual, promoting the state of meditative calm that is prized in the spiritual practices of India. It is also a wonderful aphrodisiac, possibly due to its fragrant similarity to the human pheromone alpha androsterol. A stable fixative for more delicate floral essences. World demand far outstrips the available supply, and true Mysore sandalwood is now rare and very difficult to find. Especially for blond men.

SPIKENARD *Nardostachys jatamansi*
Aroma: Pungent, musky, earthy

A popular perfume in the ancient world, which is no longer used in modern perfumery, spikenard was used in early Egypt and was found in King Tut's tomb, still fragrant after three thousand years, in a calcite vase. Native to the foothills and valleys of the Himalayas, it was also used by Solomon. Horace once promised Virgil fifty bottles of wine in exchange for a tiny onyx box of spikenard ointment. Used in Egypt in marriage ceremonies. Deeply relaxing aphrodisiac. Recommended for blond women.

TONKA BEAN *Dipteryx odorata*
Aroma: Warm, vanilla-like

The warm, comforting scent of tonka bean is due to the presence of coumarin. This is an aroma especially suited to the woman who wants to plumb the depths of intimacy with her lover but realizes she may have some deeply buried toxic emotions to get rid of first. Tonka bean and vanilla both facilitate the process by slowly healing and releasing rage and resentment without destroying a woman's equilibrium in the process. Especially for the blond female.

TUBEROSE *Polianthes tuberosa*
Aroma: Intensely sweet, floral

Tuberose is native to Mexico. Like jasmine, it is distinguished by its ability to continue to produce fragrance in its blossoms even after the flowers have been picked. Aztec herbalists named the flower *omixochitl*, bone flower, and exported it to the Philippines and East Indies. After journeying to Spain in the 16th century, tuberose was introduced to France and Italy, which led to its cultivation in Grasse for perfume. Aphrodisiac qualities are hinted at in its Indian name, *rat ki rani*, mistress of the night, and its first European botanical name, *Amica nocturna*, friend of the night. An important ingredient in perfumes such as White Shoulders and Chloe. Recommended for brown-haired men and women.

VANILLA *Vanilla planifolia* (dried bean of the orchid)
Aroma: Sweet, warm

If you want to turn on an older man, this is the scent to use. In a recent study, older men ranked vanilla as more sensual than any other aroma! Another native of Mexico, vanilla was used by the Aztecs to flavor chocolate, which was consumed in great quantities as an aphrodisiac and health beverage. The oleoresin blends well with sandalwood and spices and adds depth to floral blends. When combined with neroli, it is said to create a credible imitation of the scent of the sweet pea. Especially for dark-haired men.

VETIVER *Vetiveria zizanoides*
Aroma: Pungent, earthy

This is an oil that smells just like my grandma's root cellar. Known in India as "khus khus," the chemically complex, viscous essence is distilled from the root, which grows wild in the Himalayas. Once used to treat muslin being exported from India to Europe, it inspired the perfume Mousseline, in which it is an important ingredient. Sun blinds, baskets, and fans have been made of vetiver and then sprayed with water to release a cooling fragrance when warmed by the sun. Such fans were popular with Javan rulers and Haitians and later among the Creole belles of Louisiana. Vetiver's aphrodisiac reputation is due to its ability to deeply relax and refresh at the same time. It's a good oil to use when you want to bring your lover or your relationship down to earth. Recommended for brown-haired men.

YLANG-YLANG *Cananga odorata*
Aroma: Rich, sweet, floral

Because this essence is so universally accepted as the oil of choice for both female frigidity and anger, I wonder how much the former may have to do with the latter, as sexual coldness in a relationship can often be the result of repressed anger or rage. In any event, ylang-ylang is a turn-on essence for both sexes, and a deep relaxant as well. Native to Indonesia and the Philippines, the flower was discovered in 1770 in the Indonesian archipelago by a Captain d'Etchevery, though not exploited until a German sailor, Albertus Schwentger, was shipwrecked on the island of Luzon and, entranced by its fragrance, successfully distilled it. Samples of ylang-ylang oil were included in the Paris World Exhibition in 1893. Recommended for brown-haired women.

Distillation and Extraction Methods

MANY OF NATURE'S MOST SEDUCTIVE AROMAS are too delicate to survive the heat of the distillation process and must be won by less intense processes, such as solvent extraction or enfleurage.

Solvent extraction is likened to dry cleaning flowers to remove their essential oils. A solvent such as petroleum ether, which has a very low boiling point, is percolated through hermetically sealed vats of blossoms, then evaporated off under reduced pressure, leaving a "concrete," an intensely fragrant solid that contains plant waxes and pigments in addition to the essential oil. The concrete is then beaten with ethyl alcohol, which dissolves the waxes, which are then removed through a chilling and filtering process, leaving a tincture (essential oils in alcohol). The alcohol is distilled off by vacuum extraction, leaving an absolute with a full-bodied aroma. Time-consuming and expensive, this process is the only way to preserve certain delicate aromas, such as jasmine, violet, hyacinth, carnation, oakmoss, and Spanish broom.

Enfleurage is a technique that has been used for thousands of years. The ancient Egyptians are known to have used fats such as lard and tallow to kidnap some of Nature's more fleeting aromas. The process is still practiced today in Grasse to extract the aroma of the tuberose. Purified hog fat, or suet, is smeared with a spatula over both sides of a glass plate in a wooden frame. Flowers are placed by hand on top of the fat, and the plates are closely stacked to trap the aroma. After a day or two, the blossoms are dumped off and a fresh new layer of flowers is added. When the fat is fully permeated with scent, it is scraped off each of the glass panels, gently warmed, then filtered through gauze and left to cool. As in solvent extraction, the remaining mixture is then beaten for several days with ethyl alcohol. The fat is filtered out by chilling, leaving an extract of essential oil in alcohol. To create an *absolut d'enfleurage*, the alcohol is distilled off under a vacuum. An *absolut de chassis* is a lower-quality fragrance oil created by hexane extraction of the leftover blossoms after most of their essence has migrated into the fat in the first part of the process.

If you have tuberose or a jasmine bush blooming in your garden, you can try a simplified version of enfleurage at home. Get a large, glass, wide-mouth jar and coat the inside with pure, warm, unsalted lard or vegetable shortening. Fill it with dry, clean blossoms, preferably picked before the sun hits them on the day they open. Cap the jar tightly. If the weather is warm, keep it in the refrigerator. After one day (for jasmine) or two (for tuberose), dump the spent blossoms, picking out any that stick in the fat, and refill the jar with new blooms. Repeat the process for about a month, at the end of which you'll have a seductively scented cream that you can warm slightly to add in other essential oils, or use as a sensual massage cream or to moisturize hands and body. For those who prefer to use nonanimal fats for extraction, coconut oil or the natural version of petroleum jelly (a blend of vegetable fats and babassu oil) can be substituted, though they are not absorbed as well by the skin.

The most common method of producing essential oils is through *water* or *steam distillation*, or a combination of both. Essential oil-containing leaves, flowers, crushed seeds, or chopped roots are placed in a vat. In the case of steam distillation alone, steam is forced through the plant material under pressure. In water or water/steam distillation, the plant material is immersed in water or placed on a grille over the water, and heat is applied from beneath. The volatile oil is carried up and away on the steam, which is then cooled in a separate chamber. The essential oil floats atop the condensed vapor, or in the case of essential oils like clove or anise, falls to the bottom of the flask.

A variation on steam distillation that is commonly used to create spice essences is carbon dioxide, or CO_2 distillation, in which pressurized carbon dioxide gas is used in place of steam to extract the volatile oils.

Most citrus oils are obtained by *expression*, or cold pressing of the peels of fruits such as orange, lemon, tangerine, grapefruit, and bergamot. Water sprays over the peels as they are squeezed, creating a slurry of albedo (the white part between the peel and the fruit), pectin, cellulose, and essential oil. The slurry is screened and centrifuged, and fruit waxes are removed by chilling. After a final filtering, only the essential oil remains.

NINE

More Daily Esscentuals

Perfume and Massage Oil Recipes

The following recipe is based on a fragrant massage oil that was rubbed by female attendants into the just-bathed skin of the ruler of India each morning. Use it when you want your lover to feel like a king.

RAJAH'S MORNING MASSAGE BLEND

4 ounces sesame oil

8 drops jasmine

3 drops coriander

1 drop cardamom

2 drops basil

6 drops costus

3 drops pine

1 drop bay laurel

1 drop clove

CHRISTINE MALCOLM'S SEDUCTIVE SANDALWOOD PERFUME BLEND

This truly esscentual blend from the owner of Santa Fe Fragrance appeared in a recent issue of "Beyond Scents" Newsletter.

¹/₄ oz. jojoba oil
50 drops sandalwood
4 drops frankincense
2 drops myrrh
14 drops tangerine

10 drops ylang-ylang
1 drop nutmeg
14 drops cedarwood
2 drops rose
3 drops jasmine

ERECTOR SET

When your "get-up-and-go" has got up and gone, try this extra-stimulating blend.

4 oz. carrier oil
3 drops peppermint
5 drops clove
2 drops coriander

15 drops rosemary
20 drops lavender
5 drops rosewood
2 drops ginger

ANGEL WATER

Based on an 18th-century Portuguese aphrodisiac water, women once daubed this invitingly on bosoms exposed by the fashion of the time.

1 pt. orange flower water
1 pt. rose water

¹/₂ pt. myrtle water
10 drops ambrette essential oil

Blend all ingredients and shake well. Allow a week for the scents to mingle and settle, shaking daily. Keep in the refrigerator in warm weather, as the floral waters tend to be perishable. Makes a wonderful facial wash or spray and a delicate splash or perfume.

LOVE IN THE GRASS

My personal eau de cologne recipe has the usual piquant aroma, complicated by an aphrodisiac whisper of rose and clary sage.

2 drops rose	6 drops bergamot
1 drop clary sage	12 drops palmarosa
6 drops tangerine	30 ml/1 oz. high-proof vodka or Everclear
3 drops geranium	3 drops grapefruit
15 ml/¹/₂ oz. water	

Blend the essential oils and let them sit overnight to synergize. Add the combined essences to the alcohol (high-proof vodka works fine) and swish or stir gently but thoroughly to mix.

Let this mixture sit for a day or two, then add purified water. Allow to age for four to six weeks in a dark cupboard, giving it a shake whenever you think of it. Strain through a coffee filter and bottle.

Incense

THERE'S SOMETHING EROTIC and exotic about burning incense, the earliest form of aromatherapy. *Per fumum*, through smoke, is the origin of the word perfume, as volatile oils are released when fragrant materials are consumed with flame. The flame itself and the act of burning are closely associated with erotic love and passion. Lighting candles and incense ignites the romantic imagination, and they are a kind of sympathetic magic to use when you want to kindle a fire within.

Making your own incense allows you to be 100% certain of what you're burning, and that it contains no noxious chemicals or artificial perfume fragrances. This recipe is based on sawdust, which you can get from your neighborhood woodworker or handyman. Make sure the sawdust comes from untreated wood; redwood, cedar, and pine are the best. Sawdust from particle board contains formaldehyde, which defeats the whole purpose!

Sift the sawdust so that you have a fine powder. Combine **half a cup of water** with **one tablespoon plus one teaspoon of powdered gum arabic**, and stir until smooth. Mix bit by bit into **half a cup of sawdust**, until you have a sand-textured "dough" that can you can mold into a rod shape. Then add fragrancing materials, such as gum benzoin, powdered sandalwood, powdered frankincense, storax or spices, to total about 1/8 cup, or 1 ounce. Essential oils are added last. Mold the finished product into short, thin rods; or for fun, shape them as little lingams. Any longer than two inches and they're prone to breakage. To reinforce, let the rods dry slightly and insert toothpicks. Let them dry for a couple of days, then store in an airtight container. Burn in an incense burner, or set upright to light in a shallow dish of sand.

FOOD FOR THE GODS
To the sawdust mixture, add 1 ounce **gum benzoin**, 6 drops **frankincense**, 6 drops **myrrh**, 6 drops **sandalwood**, 2 drops rose or **jasmine absolute**.

MOCAILAMA'S TENT
To the sawdust mixture, add 1 tablespoon **gum benzoin**, 6 drops **ambrette**, 3 drops **rose**, 3 drops **neroli**, 3 drops **jasmine**. (Optional: you can add to this any of the following harder-to-find ingredients: 3 drops each of absolutes of **jonquil** or **narcissus**, **hyacinth**, and **carnation**, and a dropperful each of tinctures of **amber** and **musk**.)

TANTRIC TEMPLE

To the sawdust mixture, add 10 drops **patchouli** and 10 drops **ambrette**, or a whole dropperful of tincture of **musk** (in place of the ambrette), if you can find it.

KYPHI (A MUCH-SIMPLIFIED VERSION INSPIRED BY THE EGYPTIANS' FAVORITE PERFUME)

To the sawdust mixture, add 4 drops **spikenard**, 2 drops **peppermint**, 6 drops **myrrh**, 4 drops **juniper**, 8 drops **clary sage**, and a teaspoon each of **cinnamon** and ground **cardamom**, or 2 drops each of the essential oils of **cinnamon** and **cardamom**.

An even simpler way of creating incense is to buy charcoal tabs, light them, and toss on a pinch of resin or spice. **Gum benzoin, balsam of Tolu** or Peru, **frankincense, myrrh,** and **storax** burn well, as do **cloves, nutmeg, dried rosemary, thyme** or **lavender, anise seeds,** and **angelica root.** Distilled essential oils tend to volatilize too quickly in a charcoal tab's intense heat and are better used in a diffusor or ceramic light bulb ring.

Potpourri

To create your own potpourri, you'll need:

Large, airtight, opaque container for initial mixing (coffee can, canister, etc.)

Dried plant materials (see list)

Fixative (see list)

Essential oils (see list)

Pretty jars, sachets, or covered dishes to enclose the final product.

DRIED MATERIALS could include rose petals or buds from blossoms or bouquets given to you by your lover; dried fragrant herbs from your garden, such as basil, bay leaves, calendula or delphinium petals (for color), lavender, thyme, lemon verbena, marjoram, mint, rosemary, rose geranium leaves, yarrow; bits of dried rinds of citrus fruits (such as those left over from juice freshly squeezed for your lover); balsam pine needles; curls of birch bark; eucalyptus leaves; whole or ground spices such as allspice (whole), caraway seeds, cinnamon sticks, cloves, coriander seeds, nutmeg, or vanilla beans; bulk dried blossoms or herbs (untreated with fragrances) from herb stores.

FIXATIVES include gum benzoin, cedar shavings, clary sage leaves, frankincense gum resin, oakmoss, orris root, powdered sandalwood, tonka beans, vetiver root, or animal ingredients such as tinctures of ambergris, civet, or musk.

ESSENTIAL OILS include the following:
Balsam fir (blends well with cedar, rose, bay laurel)
Bay laurel (use in spicy, citrus or woody mixes)
Cedar (woody, spicy mixes, also with balsam or citruses)
Cinnamon (great with orange or citrus, also woody blends)
Frankincense (with spice, citrus or rose-dominated mixtures)
Geranium (florals, or to add fragrance to dried rose petal blends)
Jasmine (floral blends, powerful with rose)
Lavender (also good with rose and floral mixes)
Lemon (goes well with orange, bay, spices, woody blends)
Orange (fruity, spicy, woody blends)
Neroli (powerful with orange and spice, also woody)
Rose (beautiful with almost any blend, especially rose, or rose/lavender/cedar mix)
Sandalwood (woods, spices, florals such as jasmine, rose, and neroli)

MIXING POTPOURRI: If you're improvising, start with a little bit of each ingredient to get an idea of how they go together, both visually and for fragrance (mistakes are less costly this way, and easier to correct). Start with dry ingredients, and when you've got that part the way you want it, add your essential oils a drop at a time until you've got a delicious aroma.

A good basic formula to follow for improvisations is this: to every five cups of dried leaves, flowers, or rinds, add two and a half tablespoons of fixative, one tablespoon of spices (if you're using them), and three to ten drops of essential oil.

Then fill your aging container (air- and light-proof coffee can, jar, or canister) no more than two-thirds full. Keep the container closed for two to ten weeks, shaking daily, until the fragrance matures. Then package it in small wooden boxes, porcelain cups or sugar bowls, candy dishes, apothecary jars, or baskets. (Metal and plastic containers are usually not good choices, because they react with the essential oils.) If your potpourri loses its aroma, return it to the aging container, add a few more drops of essential oil (record your blends if you want to repeat the same aroma twice) and allow to age, again shaking daily.

You can also package your finer-textured potpourri in sachets or small pillows to be placed in drawers or among the pillows on the bed. Natural fabrics such as silk, muslin, burlap, lace, or wool work best. Simply cut two matching pieces in the shape you desire (square, rectangle, heart, circle) and sew together, leaving an opening of a few inches to turn the fabric out and insert the potpourri. After stuffing, hand-sew shut. Squeeze the sachet or pillow in your hand to release more fragrance.

LOVERS' POTPOURRI: Don't throw away those thoughtful lovers' gifts of roses or bouquets! When they've passed their prime, spread the blossoms or petals to air-dry in the kitchen. (I put mine on a cookie sheet covered with white paper, then after a few days collect the dried materials in a tightly closed jar kept in a cupboard, out of the light.) You can also dry bits of orange rind from the fresh-squeezed juice you shared together at breakfast, or lemon rind from fresh lemonade on a summer's afternoon, or cinnamon sticks from a warm mug of cocoa you snuggled over together one cold winter night. Fragrant leaves or herbs picked on a hike up a mountain or along a lake or ocean shore, wildflowers from a spring picnic . . . you get the idea. It's more than a potpourri; it's a fragrant record of your love. The longer you're together, the more interesting it becomes, and it makes a really lovely gift.

ARABIAN NIGHTS

A bedside blend, exotic, seductive, and evocative of Mocailama's tent.

1 cup dried rose petals or buds
1/4 cup myrrh
2 tbsp. cloves
2 tbsp. star anise
2 drops jasmine absolute
2 drops rose essence or absolute

1/2 cup cinnamon sticks (broken up)
1/4 cup dried jasmine blossoms
2 tbsp. cardamom seeds
2 tbsp. cedar shavings or
   sandalwood chips
2 drops cedar or sandalwood
   essence

TRUE LOVE

This is a beautiful, richly scented blend to display in the bedroom, or to make into love pillows for the bed.

1 cup dried lavender blossoms
1/2 cup dried delphinium blossoms
3 drops lavender essential oil

1 cup dried rose petals (or rosebuds)
2 tbsp. orris root chips
3 drops rose essence or absolute
   (or geranium)

KAMA'S GARDEN

What I imagine the flower-tipped arrows of India's love god to smell like! For use in a sachet or love pillow, use powdered sandalwood rather than chips.

2 cups dried patchouli leaves
1/2 cup sandalwood chips
2 drops rose geranium essence
6 drops orange

1/2 cup dried rose petals
2 tbsp. dried orange peel
2 drops patchouli

Food For Love: Aphrodisiac Recipes

One cannot think well, love well, sleep well, if one has not dined well.
VIRGINIA WOOLF

BAKED TROUT FOR TWO WITH FENNEL AND ORANGE

Fish and fennel were sacred to Aphrodite, whose name is the root of the word aphrodisiac. Oranges have been associated with love ever since Jupiter gave Juno an orange on their wedding day. Black pepper is a libido stimulator, and wine is sacred to Dionysus, one of Aphrodite's lovers.

1 oz. butter
1/2 tsp. fennel seeds
1 1/4 cups sweet vermouth
Sprigs of fresh fennel

2 medium rainbow trout, cleaned
2 oranges
Salt and freshly ground pepper

Preheat the oven to 400 degrees. Butter a shallow ovenproof dish and place the fish inside. Dot with butter and sprinkle with fennel seeds. Cut thin strips of orange rind and scatter over the fish. Squeeze the oranges over the fish, then add the vermouth. Season with salt and pepper. Cover tightly with foil and bake 25 minutes, until fish flakes easily. Serve with pan juices, garnish with fresh fennel sprigs, and top with a pat of chilled herbed butter.

MEDITERRANEAN LOVE SOUP

Fennel is considered a potent aphrodisiac in Italy and Greece.

1 oz. butter
1 large onion, chopped
2 cups milk
2 egg yolks
Salt and pepper

4 bulbs Florence fennel, sliced
4 cups vegetable stock
1 bay leaf
½ cup light cream

Melt butter in a large saucepan. Saute fennel and onion until soft, but do not brown. Add stock, milk, bay leaf, salt, and pepper. Bring to a boil, cover and simmer for 30 minutes.

Remove bay leaf and strain soup through a sieve. Mix the eggs and cream together in a bowl. Whisk in half a cup of the strained soup. Add to soup in pot, being careful not to boil to prevent curdling. Garnish with fennel sprigs.

LOVE SALAD

Fresh mixed greens, such as arugula, baby lettuce, endive, and radicchio

1 tbsp. finely chopped fennel stalk (optional)
1 tbsp. chopped parsley
1 tbsp. chopped cucumber
Sweet violet or pansy flowers, or fresh pink rose petals

Toss the first four ingredients with Love Dressing, then garnish with fresh flowers.

LOVE DRESSING

³/4 cup walnut oil
¹/4 cup fresh lemon juice
3 tbsp. rose water
Salt and freshly ground pepper

Whisk first three ingredients together and season to taste.

PASSIONATE PESTO

Basil was noted by the English herbalist Culpeper to "cure the insufficiency of Venus" and was sacred to the Haitian love goddess Erzuli. The plant is also used as a love charm by Italian girls.

2 handful fresh basil leaves
¹/4 cup pine nuts
¹/2 cup olive oil
1 lb. cooked and drained pasta

2 cloves of garlic, chopped or crushed
¹/2 cup parmesan cheese
Salt and pepper

Blend basil leaves, pine nuts, and parmesan in a blender or food processor, slowly dribbling in the olive oil. Add salt and pepper to taste. Serve with pasta, green salad, and a crusty herbed bread.

GINGER YONIS

Ginger has been praised as an aphrodisiac among Chinese, Turkish, Indian and Arabian doctors and lovers. With their suggestive shape and libido-stirring spices, these make a wonderful late-night, or between-rounds-of-love-making snack!

1 $\frac{1}{2}$ sticks sweet, soft butter
1 cup packed dark brown sugar
$\frac{1}{4}$ cup molasses
1 egg
2 $\frac{1}{4}$ cups unbleached all-purpose flour
1 tsp. ground ginger
$\frac{1}{2}$ tsp. cinnamon
Pinch cardamom
2 tsp. baking soda
$\frac{1}{2}$ tsp. salt
1 $\frac{1}{2}$ tbsp. finely chopped fresh ginger root
$\frac{1}{2}$ cup finely chopped crystallized ginger

In a large bowl, cream butter and brown sugar, then beat in molasses followed by egg. Sift together dry ingredients in a separate bowl, then stir into butter mixture with a wooden spoon. Add both chopped gingers and mix well. Cover the dough and put it in the refrigerator overnight. Preheat oven to 350 degrees. Roll bits of dough into one-inch balls and place two inches apart on greased cookie sheets. Use the blunt end of a butter knife to press an indentation into the middle of the dough balls, flattening slightly. Bake 10 minutes, or until browned. Remove to wire racks and cool. 3–4 dozen yonis.

CARROT AND GINGER LIBIDO SOUP

Carrots were called "philtron" by the Greeks, meaning "to love," and were the ultimate in pre-passion dining. Arabian women cooked them in milk spiced with cardamom to enhance their aphrodisiac effect.

$^3/_4$ stick unsalted butter
1 large yellow onion, chopped
$^1/_4$ cup finely chopped fresh ginger root
3 cloves garlic, minced
7 cups chicken stock
1 cup dry white wine
1 $^1/_2$ pound carrots, peeled, cut in $^1/_2$-inch slices
2 tbsp. fresh lemon juice
Pinch curry powder
Salt and freshly ground pepper to taste
Snipped fresh chives or parsley (garnish)

Melt butter in large stock pot. Add onion, ginger, and garlic, and saute for 15 to 20 minutes. Add stock, wine, carrots. Heat to boiling, then reduce to simmer and cook uncovered until the carrots are tender, about 45 minutes. Puree soup in a blender and return to pot. Season with lemon juice, curry powder, salt, and pepper. Sprinkle with chives or parsley. Serve hot or cold.

SPARKLING ELDERFLOWER WINE

An old English country tradition states that if a man and a woman drink elderflower wine together, they'll be married within the year.

1 gal. water

1 lemon

2 tbsp. white wine vinegar

3 ½ cups sugar

4 large elderflower heads

Warm some of the water and dissolve the sugar into it. Squeeze the juice out of the lemon and cut the rind into strips, discarding the rest. Put the flowers into a gallon jar or jug, add the lemon rind, sugar water, rest of the water, and vinegar. Stir, cover, and let sit for 4 to 5 days. Then strain the liquid into bottles with screw-on tops. In 6 to 10 days it should be effervescent. (The yeast is in the pollen, so make sure the flowers are picked on a dry, sunny day just after they've opened.)

LOVERS' LIQUEUR

Roses for the heart, spices for the heat of passion, sugar for sweetness, and alcohol for the release of inhibitions . . . the rest is up to you!

1 qt. brandy or vodka

2 cloves

2 cups strongly scented red Rose petals with white heels removed

1 cinnamon stick

1 cup sugar

Put all ingredients except sugar into a tightly closing glass jug or jar. Put in a sunny window or next to a warm stove or heater, and leave for a month. Then filter (coffee filters work fine!), add sugar, and decant in beautiful corked glass bottles.

ROSE WINE

Take three roses, white, pink and red. Wear them
next to your heart for three days. Steep them in wine
for three days more, then give to your lover.
When he drinks, he will be yours forever.

—GERMAN LOVE CHARM

Or, to make it even simpler:

1 part white wine
1 part rose water
1 part sparkling (unflavored) water

Mix in a large, chilled glass pitcher. Sprinkle in rose petals if desired. Fill
goblets with shaved ice or cubes, then pour and serve. A nonalcoholic
version can be made using rose syrup (available at Middle Eastern specialty
food stores), about a teaspoon to a cup of sparkling water.

EAST INDIAN LOVE PUDDING

An aphrodisiac dessert.

1 cup blanched almonds	1 cup sugar
3/4 cup quick-cooking farina	2 tbsp. butter or margarine
2 tbsp. rosewater	3/4 cup seedless raisins
1/2 tsp. each ground nutmeg and cardamom	4 cups milk

Brown almonds in butter. Add raisins and saute slightly. Heat milk with
sugar in saucepan. Stir in farina and cook until thickened, stirring fre-
quently. Remove from heat and add flavoring and spices. Pour ingredients

into a blender and mix. Pour into serving dish and top with reserved almonds and raisins. Serve warm. Makes 6 servings.

ROSEWATER LASSI

A delicious, nonalcoholic, refreshing, and aphrodisiac drink.

3 parts pure water, room temperature
1 part yogurt
Raw sugar or honey to taste
Bulgarian rose water (about 1 tbsp. or to taste)
Pinch of cardamom

Pour ingredients into a blender and mix thoroughly.

POACHED FRUIT

These three fruits have long served as goddess food and symbols and make a light, simple, and elegant dessert or late-night snack.

Light sugar syrup
Fresh halved apricot, fig, or peach

Poach the apricot or peach halves lightly in the syrup, then dust with a tiny pinch of cinnamon or clove. Poach fig halves with a few strips of lemon rind and a bit of ginger, then add a dollop of vanilla-flavored cream. Perfectly ripe fresh apricots, peaches, and figs are also very sexy and flavorful all by their juicy sweet selves.

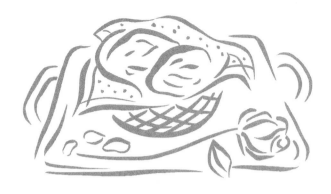

ROSE PETAL LOVE SCONES

These wonderful scones are perfect to bake and enjoy on a lazy morning after an esscentual night of love. Delicious as a light breakfast with tea or coffee. Or serve with eggs, fresh fruit, and freshly squeezed juice.

2 ¼ cups unbleached white flour
4 tbsp. unsalted butter
2 tsp. sugar
⅓ cup shelled pistachios, toasted and ground
³/₄ tsp. salt
1 cup cream
2 tsp. baking powder
1 tsp. rosewater
¹/₂ tsp. baking soda
2 to 3 pinches cinnamon
A handful of rose petals, rinsed and dried, with white heels removed

Preheat the oven to 425 degrees. In a large mixing bowl, sift together the dry ingredients and cut in the butter, pastry style, until it reaches a coarse, mealy consistency. Add pistachios. Mix the rose water into the cream. Shred the rose petals and add to the cream mixture, then stir into the dry ingredients. Drop by heaping tablespoonsful onto ungreased baking sheet. Bake 10–12 minutes, until golden brown.

ICING: Combine 1 cup confectioner's sugar, 1 tbsp. rose jelly (or red currant jelly to which $^1/_2$ tsp. rose water has been added), and 2 tsp. water. Whisk until smooth. While scones are still warm (but not hot) drizzle with icing and serve immediately. To prepare the day before, cool completely and store in airtight container. Wrap in foil and reheat for 10 to 15 minutes at 325 degrees, then frost, or serve with lightly whipped cream and rose jelly.

Love Bouquets

YOUNG GIRLS "BLOSSOM" BEFORE THEY RIPEN into womanhood, civilizations "flower," love "blooms." Flowers are a plant's way of indicating sexual readiness and maturity, which may explain why we use them so extensively in courtship and romance. During the Elizabethan and Victorian eras, lovers communicated in a language of flowers, each blossom given as a message of romantic interest, acceptance, or rejection. This custom actually started with the ancient Greeks, who sent each other telegrams in the form of bouquets and garlands of flowers, each of which had a particular meaning. The Chinese, Assyrians, Egyptians, and Indians also used "flower language" as a form of symbolic communication.

The fragrances of the following flowers are the "fresh-on-the-stem" versions of aphrodisiac essential oils and can be used for their effects when the essences you're seeking are unavailable or out of reach. Create a love bouquet based on what's available in your garden or at the florist, choosing flowers that represent the qualities you most want to encourage in your love relationship. The flowers can be given as a gift, arranged in a bedroom or throughout the house, or placed on a desk or in an office as a subtle reminder of you during your lover's workday. In addition to the beauty and elegance of their fragrances, the voluptuous forms and colors of these flowers are a subliminal encouragement to amorous thoughts and feelings.

APPLE BLOSSOM: *Love and comfort.*
Bring in blossoming branches to ease loneliness and the bumps and bruises of passionate love. In the biblical Song of Songs, Solomon's lover comforts herself with apples and the fragrance of the blooming orchards. During World War II, many a homesick and lovelorn American soldier had his sentiments expressed in a popular love song that promised, "I'll Be with You in Apple Blossom Time." (Apple and apple blossom are not available as essential oils or absolutes. "Green apple" is a synthetic perfume fragrance, as is "apple spice.")

CARNATION: *Pure love and constancy.*
Red carnations usually have the best fragrance. Give a carnation corsage or boutonnière to a lover who must travel without you, or have a bouquet waiting in the hotel room. (Carnation absolute is rare but possible to find.)

FREESIA: *Peaceful and secure love.*
The light, sweet fragrance of this spring flower banishes doubts and dissolves relationship tensions resulting from insecurity. (Not available as an essential oil or absolute.)

GARDENIA: *To increase love.*
The powerful fragrance of this flower spreads and magnifies love anywhere it's placed. (Not available as an essential oil or absolute.)

GERANIUM: *Comfort.*

A good flower for the process of recovery following a disagreement or rift in a love relationship. The fragrance is actually in the leaves, which give off more scent when bruised or rubbed between the fingers. (Readily available as an essential oil.)

HYACINTH: *Grief, love, peaceful sleep.*

Apollo had his friend Hyacinth changed into this flower after the boy was killed by an errant discus blown off course by the jealous West Wind. This is a scent to soothe a broken heart, to attract new love, and to promote sweet dreams. (Rare and costly, available as an absolute.)

JASMINE: *Sexual love, amiability.*

Roy Genders, in his book *Perfume through the Ages*, says that "the scent of the white jasmine can transform a woman into a nymphomaniac after the slightest inhalation and the tuberose has a similar effect on some women." Men and women both seem to be easily aroused by jasmine's sexy aroma. Dreams in which jasmine appears are lucky for lovers. (Available as an absolute.)

LAVENDER: *Spiritual love, true love.*

Not as sexy or heady a fragrance as jasmine or rose, the delicate scent of lavender expresses high aspirations for a love that will endure. (Available as an essential oil.)

LILAC: *Beginning love.*

The delicacy of form of the many tiny blossoms is compared to the myriad sweet and delicate emotions lovers feel at the beginning of a romance. Lilac was once thought to drive away ghosts. The 16th century herbalist Gerard described its fragrance as "troubling the head in a strange manner, and exciting the sexual instincts." (Like jasmine, tuberose, and narcissus, contains indole.) Fill the house with sprays of lilac at the start of a new love to banish the "ghosts" of old love relationships. (Not available as an essential oil or absolute.)

MADONNA LILY: *Purity, chastity.*
This is the flower to put in a bedroom arrangement when refraining from sexual involvement in a developing relationship, or to encourage constancy while your lover is away. Dreaming of lilies in bloom foretells marriage, happiness, and prosperity. Lily was sacred to Aphrodite and was associated with Lilith and Juno. (Not available as an essential oil or absolute.)

MAGNOLIA: *Giving and receiving love.*
Associated in the United States with the charm of the Southern belle, the magnolia is also a symbol of feminine beauty in China. Its rich fragrance improves the flow of love in both directions, giving and receiving. (Not available as an essential oil or absolute.)

MIMOSA: *Sensitivity.*
If your lover is overly sensitive, or if s/he runs roughshod over your feelings and finer sensibilities, try encouraging a little tenderness with the delicate perfume of this sensitive flower. (Not available as an essential oil or absolute.)

NARCISSUS: *Attentive love, aphrodisiac.*
According to Greek myth, this flower was created by Zeus to help his lovesick brother Pluto attract the attention of the maiden Persephone long enough to capture her and take her to the underworld. Thus the intoxicating aroma of narcissus is employed to attract a new love, or to pique the wandering attention of an existing lover. (Rare, but available as an absolute.)

ORANGE FLOWER: *Long-term love.*
Jupiter gave his bride, Juno, an orange at their marriage, and the flower has been used in bridal bouquets ever since. (Available as neroli essential oil or orange flower absolute.)

PLUMERIA: *Peaceful love.*
Native to Mexico, this flower is cultivated in the South Pacific and is popular for use in Hawaiian leis. Its light, lemony fragrance lifts heavy moods and dark imaginings, thereby promoting security and contentment in love. (Not available as an essential oil or absolute.)

ROSE: *Harmonious and patient love, discretion.*
Fill the house with roses to calm domestic strife or to slow down a relationship that's moving too fast. In ancient Rome, a rose fastened to the ceiling told partygoers that nothing happening in the room should be spoken of outside it, giving the rose the additional attribute of discretion. Dreams of roses portend joy, happiness, and a happy marriage. (Available as an essential oil and absolute.)

SPIDER LILY: *Love and peace.*
In numerology, six is the number of love and harmony, and this fragrant, six-petaled native of the peace-loving Hawaiian Islands gives forth a magical aroma that is tuned to the spirit of the place in which it grows. (Not available as an essential oil or absolute.)

STEPHANOTIS: *Love and peace, marital harmony.*
Another Hawaiian flower, actually native to Madagascar, used traditionally as a wedding bouquet flower. The sweet fragrance banishes domestic discord and encourages love of self and others. (Not available as an essential oil or absolute.)

TUBEROSE: *Peace and love, emotional control.*

When passions get out of hand, tuberose helps to calm raging emotions. Because, like jasmine, the flowers continue to produce scent even after they're picked, and because their aroma is stronger after sundown, tuberose is known in India as *ratki rani*, or Queen of the Night. The fragrance can be very intense. Women especially respond to it as an aphrodisiac, in which case it has been used by both Easterners and Westerners. This is another Hawaiian lei flower. (The absolute is available in the perfume trade, but is very rare and costly.)

WATER LILY (aka lotus): *Love, spirituality, happiness.*

Revered since ancient times, this flower was sacred to the ancient Egyptians and Greeks as a symbol of beauty and eloquence. In India and China, it is a symbol of the Buddha and of the unfolding process of spiritual enlightenment. It is the emblem of Paradise in Japan. Some varieties are fragrant. The flower is especially beautiful when displayed floating in a bowl of water or when growing on the surface of a garden pond, where lovers can meditate on its beauty and their own loving process of unfoldment. (Not available as an essential oil or absolute, although lotus can be found in the form of an "attar.")

VIOLET: *Humility and faithfulness.*

Violet tames the raging ego, that part of us that wants to control everything and that can easily destroy an otherwise loving relationship. Violets growing wild in the United States are generally not fragrant, but delicately scented European Parma violets are occasionally available. In ancient Greece, women rubbed an oil of violets all over their bodies before sexual union. The 13th-century occultist Albertus Magnus claimed that violets gathered during the last quarter of the moon are "love-producing," or aphrodisiac. On his way into exile, Napoleon stopped at his ex-wife Josephine's grave and plucked some of the Parma violets that were growing there.

The former emperor kept the dried flowers in a locket around his neck until he died a few years later. (There is some disagreement about the authenticity of violet absolute, which is rare at best. There is an essential oil available that is distilled from the leaves, but it doesn't smell like the violet flower.)

WHITE GINGER: *Purification, love and peace.*
This native of India still grows wild in some remote areas of Hawaii. Its delightful aroma clears the air and uplifts a room's atmosphere, especially after a lovers' quarrel or disagreement. (Not available as an essential oil or absolute. If you encounter an "aromatherapy" product using white ginger oil, it actually contains a synthetic perfume oil and is not true aromatherapy.)

YARROW: *Love and courage.*
Use yarrow as part of a bouquet to banish doubts and fears of intimacy, and to give the courage to love freely and fully.

Afterword

They are not long, the days of wine and roses:
Out of a misty dream
Our path emerges for a while, then closes
Within a dream.

ERNEST DOWSON

LOVE IS A WONDERFUL THING. Fragile as butterfly wings and hummingbird hearts (used in a Creole love charm) yet enduring as the oak (believed by the Greeks to be the first mother of men), love persists and flourishes as a shining possibility for each and every one of us. Love is the true currency of life, the wisest investment, and perhaps the only thing you really can take with you when you go. And so I encourage you to

Live! Love! Enjoy!

Safety Information and Resources

THE OILS SUGGESTED FOR USE in this book are generally recognized as safe to use in accordance with specified instructions in the appropriate dilutions (see recommended dilutions in chapter 2). There are more than 200 essential oils currently available in the marketplace, the bulk of which are used by the flavoring, fragrancing, and pharmaceutical industries. Not all of these essential oils are suitable to use for aromatherapeutic purposes. NEVER use an essential oil without being fully knowledgeable about its purity, its purpose, its safety, and its proper application.

I do not advocate the internal usage of essential oils or aromatherapy products due to possible damage to internal organs as a result of improper or extended use. High internal dosages of certain essential oils can cause convulsions, kidney and liver damage, miscarriage, and, with certain toxic oils, death. Keep your oils properly labeled and stored out of the reach of children. Use only pure, aromatherapy-grade essential oils sold by reputable suppliers such as those listed in the Resource Guide at the end of this book.

The following oils are TOXIC and should never be used for aromatherapy:

Boldo	Mustard	Horseradish	Wormseed
Mugwort	Pennyroyal	Calamus	Thuja
Wormwood	Bitter almond	Savin tansy	Savory
Rue	Wintergreen	Cornmint	Camphor
Ajowan	Buchu	Sassafras	

In addition to the oils listed above, the following oils should also be avoided during pregnancy:

Basil	Bay laurel	Clove	Myrrh birch
Origanum	Marjoram	Tarragon	Thyme

The following oils are very irritating to the skin and should not be used in bath or massage:

Cassia	Origanum

The following oils are potentially irritating to mucous membranes, such as the mouth, respiratory tract, and genitourinary tract. Use only a drop or two diluted in a carrier, and discontinue using these oils in bath or massage if irritation results.

Clove	Cinnamon	Thyme	Peppermint
Spearmint	Bay laurel		

The following oils are phototoxic and can cause permanent pigment discoloration if applied to the skin before exposure to the sun:

Bergamot (except for bergapteneless)

Lemon	Lime	Bitter orange	Angelica
Cumin	Opoponax	Verbena	

The following oils should be used sparingly to prevent dermal sensitization in highly sensitive individuals. If irritation occurs, discontinue use.

Citronella	Geranium (Reunion)	Ginger litsea
Cubeba	Pine (dwarf or Scotch)	Terebinth
Peru balsam	Benzoin resinoid	Bay laurel
Costus	Ylang-ylang	

Essential Oils

The following are reputable suppliers of essential oils. Call for catalogs and ordering information, or for a store location near you.

Aroma Vera 1-800-669-9514

Time Laboratories 1-208-232-5250

Carrier Oils

Most carrier oils can be easily found in your local grocery or health food store.

Essential Oil Products

JUST BECAUSE IT SAYS "AROMATHERAPY" on the label is no guarantee that you're getting a product made with authentic essential oils. The following companies can be relied upon to supply quality products using pure essential oils. Look for them in your local health food store or bath and body boutique, or call the company to find a retail location near you.

Aromaland 1-800-933-5267
Essential Oil Blends and Diffusers

Aroma Vera 1-800-669-9514
Essential Oils, Aromatherapy Bath and Beauty Products

Carol Corio Quality of Life Associates 1-800-688-8343
Aromatherapy Diffusers and Products

Essential Aromatics 1-805-640-1300
Aromatherapy Candles, Bath Salts, Massage Oils, hand-crafted in Ojai, California

Mon Jardinet 1-212-877-3044
Aromatherapy Bath and Body Care Products

Original Swiss Aromatics 1-415-479-9121
Essential Oils, Aromatherapy Bath, Beauty and Massage Products

Time Laboratories 1-208-232-5250
Essential Oils and Aromatherapy Products

Further Education

Pacific Institute of Aromatherapy 1-415-479-9121
Dr. Kurt Schnaubelt, Certification and Correspondence Courses